WATCH FOR A CLOUD OF DUST

Memories of a Dixie Veterinarian

by John E. McCormack, D.V.M.

To The Rineharts —
With my best
Wishes. Sincerely
John McCormack
7/22/86 —

W. D. Hoard & Sons Company
Fort Atkinson, Wisconsin

Introduction

The title of this book, Watch for a Cloud of Dust, came about because of a former employer of Dr. McCormack, Dr. Max Foreman. Dr. Foreman, an enthusiastic and excellent veterinarian, worked at a fast pace and believed in making farm calls quickly.

"Hang up the telephone and watch for a cloud of dust!" he often loudly exclaimed to a client requesting emergency service, before he sprinted to his truck and raced to the farm.

Dr. John started writing short newsletter articles on livestock health when he was a member of the Georgia Extension Service staff. His belief that all farmers and veterinarians have similar humorous experiences led to his stories in HOARD'S DAIRYMAN magazine about Carney Sam Jenkins, a calf named Meathead and Sherman the bull. He believes that we all need to learn how to laugh at ourselves occasionally.

Contents

iv

Dedicated to my father, Edward McCormack, and to the memory of my mother, Martha Stevenson McCormack. They taught by example, perserverance, tolerance, and love of the land.

1

A veterinarian needs a case like Brownie

THE voice on the two-way radio crackled out the late night message into the warmth of the pickup cab.

"Fresh cow down, bloated, prolapsed uterus. They want you as soon as possible!"

As my wife's voice slowly recited directions to the scene of the emergency, I wondered aloud if this would be a DOA (dead on arrival) trip, and if not, which one of the problems I should attack first. Should I sit the cow up and see if she debloated by belching or should I pass a stomach tube or should I just trocarize.

It would be tough trying to put a prolapse back into a down and bloated cow. Perhaps I should get some calcium into her immediately, if she had milk fever, and then concern myself with the secondary problems. To make matters worse, it was one of those bitter cold and pitch black nights.

Roaring down the gravel road, I spotted the light in the driveway too late and ran past the turn. As I reversed the vehicle, I could see someone running toward the road, frantically waving a kerosene lantern. As I drew closer, I realized that the lantern waver was a young woman. Two little boys were at her side hanging onto her tattered coat-tail, and both were crying.

Family milk cow . . .

"Brownie's dyin'!" one of them blurted out, between sobs.

A quick history revealed that Brownie, the family milk cow, had come up with a fine heifer calf that morning. Late that afternoon they observed nothing amiss, but when she was seen about 9 p.m., she was down.

As my flashlight beamed over the prostrate bovine figure, I first thought she was beyond help. She was dangerously rotund from bloat and from her rear parts there seemed to flow an endless quantity of reddish-brown inside out uterus which blended in with the mud.

Turning my attention to her head, I discovered that she did have an eye wink reflex and was breathing. Assuming milk fever, I delayed any further exam and hustled to the truck for stomach tube, warm calcium, IV set and needle.

As the three family members watched helplessly, I passed the stomach tube, relieved the gas and started IV calcium.

"Could you two young doctors hold this bottle for me while I work on Brownie?" I asked.

Both boys charged to help. As they both held the calcium bottle, I stripped off my shirt and attempted to clean up the prolapse as best I could. Cleaning a mud-,blood-, and debris-covered prolapsed uterus is not easy, as anyone who has tried it can attest.

There is never enough water or clean drapes or old raincoats or whatever. But as the boys regulated the calcium flow with my instructions, I eventually got the red mass cleaned. Stuffing it back in and getting it inverted properly took a lot of straining, pushing and shoving.

After finishing, we sat Brownie up and she belched off more gas, urinated and passed manure. The boys had gone to the spring and fetched two pails of water which I used to wash the icicles off my arms.

As I washed, the wife explained that her husband worked the night shift at the textile mill and tried to farm a little on the side during the daytime. Brownie was their only cow and she furnished milk for not only their family but for relatives down the road, as well. Everyone had plenty of milk to drink and she also made butter. The family was poor and, thus, Brownie was important to them.

A quick prayer . . .

As I stepped back through the gate to see if Brownie could get up, I closed my eyes and said a quick prayer. This family needed this cow! I stuck my knees into her ribs and yelled. Nothing happened. A second try was equally unsuccessful. On the third try, she shakily got up on her knees and rear end, like cows do, and rested there briefly before standing the rest of the way up.

As we watched her with lantern and flashlight, she started cautiously taking some steps toward the water bucket. She drank, then walked with confidence toward the hay rack. She looked great at the moment. I just hoped that she didn't relapse.

After some discussion about milking out, feeding and housing, I said goodbye and started for the truck. Suddenly, the older of the two boys rushed up, hugged my leg and said, "Thanks, Mister, for makin' Brownie well!"

Driving home that night I had this exuberant feeling of having done something good and important. I was a fairly new graduate and had not experienced many situations like this. It was good to be able to help an animal and its owner!

I passed that farm many times after that night. If I saw the boys playing in the yard, I would honk the horn and they would rush to the edge of the road and wave until I was around the curve and out of sight. I also saw Brownie grazing contentedly in the small pasture beside the road and each time I remembered that cold night, struggling with her life. Then I'd have that good feeling again. As far as I know, Brownie was never sick again.

Every veterinarian needs a case like this occasionally to recharge his or her mental batteries. This case happened long ago; yet, I remember it like it was yesterday. By saving this cow, I helped this family. This cow was important to the diet of those boys and their cousins.

The practice of veterinary medicine has changed a great deal over the years. Fortunately, we don't have as many of these type cases as we once did. Milk fever can be better controlled through dry cow nutrition so it is not the problem it was.

We still treat sick animals, but perhaps veterinarians make a greater contribution today by assisting dairymen in preventing diseases, improving reproductive efficiency and in working with other service people to insure healthy herds. Still, I think I wanted to become a farm veterinarian because of the Brownies of the world.

2

I remember the county's first C-section

IT WAS about 3 p.m. Easter Sunday when the phone rang. Even though I was snoozing peacefully on the couch, I was relieved to hear the jingle of Ma Bell, since the suspense finally was lifted. Now I could get on with the work at hand and get it done.

It was Mr. Kent Radloff on the other end of the line. He was a tough, independent type, just like most of my farmer clients. He didn't mince words; nor did he like to call the cow doctor without due cause. This was due cause!

"Doc, I need you to come help us birth a calf," he drawled.

The key word in this brief utterance was the word "us." What this meant was that all the neighbors had tried, as had all the kinfolks, and even two surprised drunks driving down the gravel road had been flagged down and they, too, had become exhausted or given up in their first obstetrical exercise.

"How long's she been laboring, Mr. Kent?"

"Aw, just since yesterday about dinnertime," he allowed. This meant that she'd been trying to calve for at least two days. Poor beast, she'd not only been in natural misery from her labors, but also had bravely tolerated the prolonged internal gropings of well-meaning but unqualified would-be obstetricians.

"Mr. Kent, we'll probably need to do a Cesarean on that heifer," I suggested, weakly.

"What you talking 'bout, Doc?" he asked.

I had been up to Mr. Kent's place only once before, to Bang's test his 75 cows, and I knew that his knowledge of veterinary matters did not extend much beyond coal oil drenches, splitting hollow tails and smearing hog lard for rattlesnake bites. When he didn't know what a Cesarean

4

section was, I feared that I was going to have trouble.

The trip to the farm took only about 15 minutes. As I topped the hill and looked down at the farm, I could see numerous cars and pickup trucks pulled off on the road shoulder. Drawing nearer, the scene resembled a family reunion, a Methodist quarterly meeting or a goat killing. There were overalled, baseball capped farmers with hands stuffed deep into their pockets, milling about, some gazing expectantly towards town, while others were excitedly pointing their fingers towards the new vet who by now could be seen nearing the appointed scene. Several observers had secured ringside seats atop the rickety catch pen fence and they were busy adjusting great cuds of chewing tobacco into comfortable quarters inside their bulging cheeks.

As I neared the corral, a host of young junior cattlemen raced to see who would be first to drag open the halfway fallen down barbed wire gap.

After parking and pulling clean white coveralls over my street clothes, I made my way over to the patient, a 500-pound Angus-Hereford cross heifer. As I carried lariat, bucket, chains and calfjack, I could hear the old timers in the background.

"Ain't never seed no vetnerry with white clothes on before!" sneered one.

"I cudda pulled that calf myself if'n I'd a had them chains and that cumalong thang," offered another.

"He's a big feller awright, but if Unca Silas can't git that calf, can't nobody!" echoed another.

The heifer was in remarkably good physical and mental condition, considering what she had been through. Examination revealed a very swollen and dry vagina which contained stubs of two amputated forelegs attached to what felt like the biggest fetus ever presented in that county.

"Mr. Kent, we're gonna have to take this calf out of her side," I stated, assertively.

A hush fell over the attentive multitude. A select few had heard of such, but most were nonbelievers in such shenanigans.

"Who ever heard tell of slicin' open a cow to get a calf?" one whiskered citizen mumbled.

I could hear other comments being offered by other self-

5

acclaimed experts as Mr. Kent and I negotiated a settlement to the problem at hand. I was determined that I had to perform surgery on that heifer, and I was just as determined that she was going to survive. It was against my principles to treat cows on halves, but this one time I decided to go against my principles.

"Tell you what, Mr. Kent, we'll operate on the cow and, if she dies, you don't owe me a thin dime," I heard myself say.

"What if she lives though?"

"If she lives, you give me half interest in her and we'll sell her at the stockyard this fall."

"Hop to it, then, Doc!"

By this time, the audience was exchanging bets and greenbacks were being flashed around like a cockfight was imminent.

Putting the heifer down, the shaving, scrubbing, and anesthetizing the incision site was accomplished in short order. Making that first skin incision is always a dramatic moment — kind of like the kickoff in a football game. Continuing my incision down through the oblique muscles, I encountered the inevitable bleeders, which were carefully clamped off with forceps. Nevertheless, blood began to become more visible.

A sudden commotion caused me to turn around and look towards the fence.

"KA-WHUMP!!"

Joe Bob Jenkins had fainted at the sight of the blood and had fallen off the top board of the fence backwards! Everyone rushed to see if he was still alive, leaving me alone with my patient.

While they were administering to Joe Bob, I extracted the uterus from the abdominal cavity of the heifer and had almost finished removing the semirotten fetus when my team of assistants returned.

Bad odors get to some people and this was no exception. Suddenly, the fence was empty and bodies were streaking for the bushes with hands over mouths and with throats making gargling noises. It was as though the audience had been hit with cannisters of tear gas. Joe Bob was by now sitting up, glass eyed, in amongst a patch of pokeweed, trying to figure out what day it was and which pickup truck

6

had desensitized him.

One of my faults is an uncontrollable urge to snicker and laugh whenever surgical procedures lead to gagging and nausea by the observers. I'm sorry, I just cannot control myself. Imagine then, my condition upon seeing 20 or so boys and men heaving and harking, six or eight more trying to remain stoic but whose faces were the color of bleached-out rice, and one half-comatose, unattended zombie that was knee-walking through pokeweeds.

With tears rolling down my cheeks and my body shaking with spasms of stifled snickering, I finally, with great effort, closed the uterine incision.

Putting in the sutures always takes a long time for me. By the time I got to the skin sutures, the survivors of the nausea attack had returned for additional observation. Now I was in control of the situation. I had not gotten sick, so to them I was a really tough individual.

"Look at 'im handle them tools," one dry mouthed cowboy marveled. "He's tying knots with them little silver pliers."

"This instrument is called a needle holder, and those over there on the drape are called mosquito forceps," I lectured, as if they were first-year veterinary students.

"How many of these operations have you done, Doc?" asked one of the quicker thinkers.

"Aw, a heap!" I exclaimed, not defining the word "heap." Certainly no one wants their cow to be the first.

When the ropes were released, the heifer scrambled to her feet with enthusiasm and tried to run out the open gap.

"Look at 'er, she feels better already!" exclaimed an overalled cowboy. Most of them were on my side now.

"Probably lookin' for a place to die," drawled another one who was not convinced yet.

While cleaning the instruments at the back of my truck, I saw the animal begin to graze. Mr. Kent's frown slowly gave way to a semismile as he eased to my side.

"Doc, lemme pay you now and we'll just forget about that partnership," he said.

"Naw, why don't we just wait and sell her and I'll just take half."

"Doc, please let me just go ahead and write you a check right now," he pleaded.

As you might suspect I did "let" him pay me that day. The heifer had no complications from the surgery and did well.

An incident like this one can do wonders in building a reputation for a young veterinarian. In that little backwoods community, they are probably still telling their stories about Doc and Mr. Kent's cow. The more the story gets told, the bigger it gets!

One reason this case is so vivid in my memory is that it was the only time that I can recall when a farmer begged to pay me. I wish I had that on tape; then I could play it back for my clients now!

3

Never again will I jump a hoglot fence

I SEEM to be injury prone whenever my work leads me towards the vicinity of the hoglot.

Years ago, while employed by Dr. Max Foreman in south Alabama, I was called to check a sow that was off-feed. Being an enthusiastic fence jumper, I tried to hurdle the board fence after arriving at the farm. With bucket in one hand and drug case in the other, I came down hard on my right ankle and it buckled under the load. I can still hear the sickening sound of ligaments and tarsal bones being ripped asunder as I staggered and fell into copious quantities of gummy mud and hog manure. Writhing and wallowing in pain, I wondered for a brief instant why I hadn't decided to enter a small animal practice in Memphis.

After several minutes of grimacing and ankle-holding, it became apparent that I would not be in any condition to continue on into the hog house, search out the patient and make an examination. In addition, by then the former slim and supple ankle was grossly swollen, and my attempts to remove the Justin roughout boot were met with much difficulty, primarily in the form of excruciating pain and misery.

Eventually, the boot came off, which was good, since the ankle throbbed less after that, but within minutes its size had reached mammoth proportions. At that point, it would have had great difficulty fitting into a five-pound lard bucket.

Hobbling to the truck with the aid of a 2 by 4 scantling, I called into the office on the two-way.

"Mobile three to base, mobile three to base," I called, in a weak and pitifully shaky voice.

"Go ahead, Dr. John," Mrs. Lee replied.

"Mrs. Lee, I've broken my ankle!" I relayed. "It's swollen up real bad, and I can't put any weight on it, and it hurts really bad."

"Oh no!" she cried, "Hold tight for a minute, you poor dear."

As I eased down on the seat of the truck with my foot elevated on a case of calcium, the thought that my good friends would be arriving shortly consoled me.

I closed my eyes in a semi-faint and envisioned them all leaving the clinic in pickup trucks and four-wheel drive Jeeps, throwing gravel and kicking up great clouds of dust. I could picture them as they hurtled through the traffic light, with horns blaring and arms waving. Surely the town's one ambulance would be following close behind, and it would also be literally bolting through town with sirens wide open and with the driver bent over the steering wheel in deep driving concentration.

Without a doubt, the sheriff and the town constable would fall into the scurrying procession when they found out that good ol' Doc had really boogered up his leg.

Ah, it is great to have friends like these. Who needs a safe, white-smocked small animal practice in Memphis anyway. I felt guilty for even thinking about living anywhere else. Give me a small town anytime.

Take afternoon off . . .

The radio brought me out of my coma.

"Dr. John, are you there?"

I groaned.

"Dr. John, Dr. Foreman said to tell you that since it is already 4:30, for you to go ahead and take the rest of the afternoon off. He'll take the rest of your farm calls," she recited.

"You mean nobody's coming out here," I said in disbelief. "I'm dyin'!"

"Everybody here is tied up, Dr. John. Whitney is clipping those poodles, Dr. Foreman is in the northern part of the county right now, and Woody is breeding cows at Silver Valley Dairy," she said. "Maybe you can apply some Bag Balm on your leg and that will make it all better!"

"What!" I ranted to myself. "I'm out here all by myself, dyin' in a stinkin' hog lot, and she tells me to smear Bag

10

Balm on my ankle, and it's just five minutes from fallin' off! A lesser man would have been dead minutes ago!"

At that point, the owner of the farm finally decided to show up and see what I had to say about the sow.

"I'm sorry, Sir," I began, "but as you can see by that leg over yonder on the calcium box, I am unable to perform an examination and treat your animal. My leg is severely and probably permanently damaged."

"Does that mean you won't charge me for a call?" he asked happily.

As adrenalin surged through my boiling circulatory system, my previous feeling of affection and brotherhood suddenly turned to a feeling of infuriated rage. Looking back, I am sure that I was delirious.

With teeth clenched and eyelids narrowed, I decided to show them all that I didn't need their help. I would drive to the hospital by myself, walk in the front door dragging my leg behind me, and tell 'em to get me some help right now! And furthermore, I'd just double dog dare 'em to say one word about being covered with stinking hog manure.

The 10-mile drive into town can best be described as an ordeal. Since the truck had a manual transmission, it was very difficult to manipulate clutch, brake, and accelerator with my sound left foot. I found that if I used the 2 by 4 scantling as an accelerator-pressing device, then I could propel the vehicle. There was a lot of jumping and jerking, sudden stops and veering off the road.

But this type driving is not considered at all abnormal for large animal vets in that rural vicinity. So, when I met clients and friends on the road, they would give me a wide berth, as usual, and not even realize that the weaving and jerking truck and the panic-stricken look on my face were not normal operating procedures.

The arrival at the hospital was uneventful, except for a lot of noseholding and astonished frowns that were directed towards the smelly vet. That problem was corrected quickly by issuing the patient a blue gown with the entire back part gone out of it. Hospital gowns, by the way, are only one of the methods of humiliating upstart patients. The smelly clothes were taken out of the emergency room on a long broom handle and incinerated.

An angel of mercy appeared and stabbed my arm with a

sedative, and the next thing I knew I was being brought back into consciousness by another, quite talkative angel in the recovery area.

"That sure is a big and heavy cast that the doctor applied, isn't it," she literally shouted to her colleague, who was only inches away.

"Yep, sure is!" screamed nurse number two. "I'll bet he'll be staying inside the vet clinic for a long time working on scratchy poodles and coughing Chihuahuas!"

"Why do you say that?" I whispered slowly, groggily.

"Well, I was raised on a dairy farm," she yelled, "and I know that a vet can't get around a muddy lot with a big cast on like that."

"Well, what do you think we should have done?" asked the doctor sarcastically as he arrived on the scene.

"Looks to me like you could have just smeared some Bag Balm on it and sent him out the door," she countered.

I flopped my head back on the pillow and went to sleep.

4

"They found oil at Tater Tom Tyree's!"

I'M SO glad that country folks can have nice things, too," I remember my dad saying many years ago.

We had just visited in a farm home a pretty good distance from ours, and those people had plenty of running water, a nice bathroom furnished with those swanky, thick, store-bought towels in several colors and electric lights that were recessed in the ceiling. Up to that point, the only towels that I had ever seen were kind of a dull off-white color with the faint shadow of the numbers 3-9-6 or 6-8-4 still readable when you held them up against the light just right. They were scratchy, too, and didn't absorb much water.

I was not, nor am I now, the least bit ashamed of those towels, nor the fact that we used them for drying our hands or bodies. It's just that I have nicer ones now, and it seems like such a long time ago when we didn't have them.

It is especially gratifying to see farmers come into unexpected wealth or have good fortune, especially when those families have struggled to make ends meet by scraping out a living on rocky hillsides or marshy pastures.

Tater Tom Tyree was such an individual. He was a good, sincere and dependable man, but somehow he never could get ahead. He also was lame from a pulpwood loading accident, but he refused to let it interfere with his job.

Poorest farm in county . . .

Tater had managed to save and borrow enough money to make a down payment on the poorest farm in the county. His plan was to raise beef cattle on the 120 acres and work part-time at the filling station.

Tater's farm was one of those farms where nothing seemed to grow very well. The grass never was as green and pretty as the neighboring farms, there was never enough water and the cattle just never seemed to do well on that place. Nevertheless, he was high as a kite over having his own place, and I hoped and prayed that he would be successful.

Things went badly from the start, however. First, he used questionable judgment by going across the state line and buying 75 sale barn cows. Since brucellosis was much more widespread then than today, and the rules and regulations were not enforced well at the time, he unknowingly purchased cows that came from an infected herd. He swore the cows were "guaranteed" and were "clean," but somewhere along the line things went awry.

"Doc, these here cows are coughin' and snortin', and some of 'em are breathin' with their mouths open," he reported over the phone early one autumn morning. "What do you reckon's goin' on?"

"Tater, sounds like you've got big trouble. Shipping fever most likely," I said.

"Well, come on down here and see if you can he'p me out," he asked nervously.

It was a classical shipping fever outbreak. Today it is not in vogue to call it "shipping fever." Bovine respiratory disease is the proper term now, and I often am reminded of the correct terminology when I slip and say "shipping fever."

Many of Tater's cows and yearlings were affected, so we treated all we could catch in the old barn. Tater ran up a sizable bill with my making several 20-mile round trips, treating the sick ones and dispensing medicine for him to administer. He lost only two cows and had three or four chronics, so he and I felt like all the effort had been worth it.

Over the following month, he had numerous other herd health problems. In the winter, he had several cows abort. When we started testing for brucellosis every 30 days, we had other problems.

One day a cow came flying through the chute, only to break her neck when she hit the head catch. Naturally, he said it was his best cow.

An early spring thunderstorm killed three head that were standing under an old oak tree. Two of those were his

14

best calves, he said.

A bull was killed when he got onto the train tracks and challenged a locomotive.

Several of the Angus heifers became paralyzed while trying to deliver large calves. The previous owner had allowed the small heifers to be pasture exposed to a Charolais bull. We performed C-sections on some and had to assist several others. His bad luck never stopped.

The brucella germ that had gotten into his herd was an especially "hot" one. We were testing faithfully every 30 days, but after six months we had branded and sold half his herd and still were finding more suspects and reactors.

Although my outlook and enthusiasm for Tater's future was somewhat dimmed, he never openly exhibited any great degree of pessimism. He always believed that he eventually would have that clean and healthy herd.

Big news . . .

I first read about the big news in the local weekly paper. "Petroleum companies checking for oil in south end of county,"I remember the paper reported. The search was centered 10 miles south of town on state highway 19. Then the rumors started.

"They've found oil pure enough to put right into your crankcase down there in Tater Tyree's pasture," one report said.

"They'll be pumping $3,000 worth a day from Tater's backyard," said another.

"Tater won't git nothin' but a few dollars a day after the company and taxes git through with it," said a third.

Speculation was high about the new unexpected wealth to befall Tater and the county.

"Let's just wait and see," he said one day when I asked him about the oil deal.

He, several other men and I were working the cattle one summer day when the big event happened. His wife came to the edge of the pasture in her old Ford and started blowing the horn, waving frantically, and shouting. Tater went to her in a full sprint. After two minutes of running and about five seconds of conversing, he started jumping up and down and hollering like a little kid heading for the ice cream factory.

"They've hit it! They've hit it! It's oil! Oil!" he shouted at the top of his lungs. "I can't believe it, Doc!" he puffed and slobbered as he neared the catch pen.

Pretty soon everybody was jumping up and down, yelling and laughing. They, because of their new wealth, and me because now Tater was going to be able to pay his overdue vet bill!

I have not seen Mr. Tater Tyree in about 15 years, since I moved away from that area. I have heard, though, that his wife always has a new silver Cadillac, he always has a new four-wheel-drive pickup truck and he has a fine herd of clean and healthy purebred Angus cows. Oh yes, he also has a new house with five bathrooms.

I'm so glad that country people can have nice things!

5

Animals get into such predicaments

THE general public has no conception of what livestock owners and others, who make their living dealing with animals, experience and endure, in terms of accidents, strange happenings, or just downright ridiculous occurrences.

Just the other day, we were in the process of putting a herd of Holsteins through the parlor for Bang's and TB tests. Suddenly, a first-calf heifer came charging through, jumped over the front gate and vaulted head first over a five-foot tall barrier into the brimming full flush tank.

Everyone was agape at the flopping-around heifer while I was trying frantically to grab and protect the multitude of Bang's and TB forms, blood tubes, syringes and needles from water damage.

As she paddled vigorously and splashed around in the cold water with great authority and apparent delight, the rest of us were attempting to avoid the wet stuff while trying to figure how to get the brute out of her predicament. In just a few short seconds, she had managed to get herself hung halfway over one of the metal partitions and was lodged there with sides pooching out and tail slinging dark green water all over the previously spotless parlor.

After what seemed like several minutes of staring at each other and calling for opinions on how to proceed, someone showed up with two lariats and a halter. With great difficulty, we managed to get her haltered and the other ropes looped around her legs. We enlisted the help of every available hand on the premises and somehow rolled her up and out of the tank.

To our surprise, the heifer didn't have a single broken bone nor other visible sign of trauma. There was a small jagged, three-inch laceration on the back of her udder that we sprayed with Topazone. Later, the owner reported that she gave more milk that night than usual and he reckoned that we probably ought to make her jump back into the tank again.

Mule named Truman . . .

Another incredible accident occurred one summer on a cotton farm several years ago when a mule named Truman was spooked by a not-so-bright kid. Somehow the mule had escaped from his stall and had managed to get inside the pole barn that housed the tractor and other farm equipment. When the half-wit threw corn cobs at the beast to make him move out, the mule decided to attempt to go up and over the C Farmall all rigged up with the cultivator. His attempt was unsuccessful.

There was a half-inch rod with a cotter key in the end of it on the back part of the cultivator, and this pierced Truman's abdomen. Thus he became impaled.

"Doc, come quick! My mule's done jabbed a steel rod up in his belly and he's hung!" was the frantic message that I received over the cracking and popping eight-party line telephone.

Sure enough, upon my arrival at the farm, I was surprised to see a blue nosed mule semiskewered on a C Farmall cultivator rod. He was sort of precariously balanced on the thing, with all four feet just off the ground; yet he was not struggling but was looking around at his problem as if meditating.

After several long seconds of thought, we secured a hacksaw and, with much effort and sweat, sawed the rod in half and Truman was free. But then a new problem surfaced. As he rolled slowly off the cultivator and the steel rod pulled free, it also pulled out portions of his intestines. So there he was with two feet of limp but neat intestines hanging from the jagged laceration in his body wall.

Back then, I didn't know that equines were supposed to die quickly from severe abdominal wounds. If shock doesn't kill them, peritonitis will. Nevertheless, I anesthetized him with chloral hydrate, rolled him up on his back and started to work. We cleaned all the prolapsed viscera, saturated it with Furacin, stuffed it back into the abdominal cavity and sutured the wall closed with vetafil.

Truman ate a big breakfast the next morning and didn't appear any worse for his accident except for a considerable amount of swelling underneath his belly. He was back at work in just a few weeks. For several years thereafter, I would see him at work in the cotton field or he'd just be dilly-dallying around in his pine-tree-dotted loafing lot. I am certain that if he had been a valuable high bred type equine, he would not have had a chance of survival. I still don't know why he lived.

Wild Angus bull . . .

An amusing incident involving a wild Angus bull occurred at a great southern institution of higher learning several years ago. We were trying to coax a bad-tempered bull by the name of Jughead into the Powder River squeeze chute. The chute and working pens were situated just outside the modern, glass-doored administrative offices.

As the efficient and enthusiastic secretarial staff happily typed their memos and reports inside the offices, outside a dramatic event with serious consequences was unfolding. With lighting speed, Jughead escaped the headgate and made a beeline for the series of glass doors surrounding the offices.

Do you remember the noise made when an inaccurately thrown baseball crashed through your Momma's living room window during a woman's home demonstration club meeting? Multiply this sound a hundred times and you have some conception of the racket created when Jughead made his rude and totally unexpected entrance into the office foyer.

Immediately following the sounds of a million pieces of glass shattering, from the office emitted an in-unison chorus of astonished and bewildered female shrieks and another deafening sound of cheap waiting room chairs being karate chopped under the churning dinner-plate-sized feet of an enraged ruffian.

I opened one eye just in time to see four secretaries standing on their desks holding their skirts up, as if they just had seen a 2,000-pound mouse. One second later old Jug collapsed the second glass door to the outside and quickly made an entrance onto the paved farm-to-market road. After a couple of head fakes at a horn-honking

Mercedes and a Mazda, he bashed in the left door of a Toyota pickup.

Jughead finally was corralled after we turned out classes and enlisted several cowboys.

Working with livestock certainly never becomes dull since there is always something new.

Excuse me, I have to go help get a cow out of a well!

6

Good stallside manner

THE other day several faculty members were conversing about a particular senior veterinary student in their classes.

"He's really sharp," one volunteered. "He knows more medicine than any student I've ever taught."

"That's true," argued another teacher, "but his stallside manner leaves a lot to be desired."

"What difference does that make?" replied the first. "What counts is if he can practice quality medicine."

"That's where you are dead wrong," allowed the second. "He can be the best medicine man in the state and still fail at practice if he can't get along with farmers."

For many years I have observed that the best student often does not make the best practicing veterinarian. Often it is the average, even below average student, grade-wise, who develops into the most effective and most respected practitioner. One reason may be that the less brilliant student has to study and work harder to master the difficult courses in veterinary school and he is often more humble and more tolerant of the mistakes of his fellow man. The student who always makes an A + on the examination certainly knows all the technical information but often does not do a good job in his relationship with others — especially farmers.

In my dealings with farmers, I have observed that they will utilize the services of a veterinarian more frequently if they "like" that particular person. They use that practitioner because he or she not only is concerned about the health of their livestock, but also is concerned about the farmer's crops, his family or his future. Another veterinarian might be a "better" practitioner but doesn't have that special human touch.

I once rode with a veterinarian for a time who was a master at public relations or good stallside manner. While at the farm, he would inquire sincerely about the corn crop, how Junior was doing in school or whether Miss Ethel's arthritis was acting up lately. He would make a point to compliment the farmer on how clean the parlor was, how sleek the cows were or comment on the manners of the family dog. He taught me a few things about dealing with farmers who already had diagnosed hollowtail or hollowhorn in their sick cows.

"Doc, she's got the hollertail," a farmer would tell me. "I've already split her tail and put salt and pepper on it. But she still ain't right. Reckon what it is?"

Right here I used to explode!

"You dumb jerk," I'd shout. "Don't you know better'n that! There ain't no such thing as stupid hollertail. When are you ignorant people gonna learn!"

I noticed, though, after an outburst like this, that the farmer would not ask me for a return visit, even if my magic medicine had worked wonders for the cow.

My practitioner friend had a different approach, and he usually was invited back, plus the folks loaded him down with collard greens, strawberries and other delicacies.

"You know, Joe, you may just be right about hollertail. I was at a vet meeting the other day in Nashville and there's a new medicine on the market that's supposed to work on real difficult cases like this one. Would you mind if we try it on this cow? It's high, but since we're kinda using your cow as an experiment, I'll just knock a right smart off the bill. How's that?"

Of course, the farmer's reply was always in the affirmative.

That's positive stallside manner! That practitioner got the job done, too, but he approached it in a different manner. Naturally, I learned quickly from him, and now I rarely get visibly upset when faced with a farmer-diagnosed case of hollertail even though it may be the hollerbelly!

I developed a close friendship with one dairyman, primarily because of a single ridiculous incident that occurred on my first visit to his farm. We were "working" the calves and I was crouched down in the chute behind a particularly nice Holstein heifer. As I removed an extra teat, she suddenly extracted her head from the headgate, came stomping backwards over me with legs churning and hooves flying. When she finally had wiped all four feet over my new white coveralls, she trotted out into the corral with a victorious grin on her silly face.

By now the dairyman was rolling on the ground, guffawing and cracking his sides with laughter. As I spat out dirt, mud, manure and various tooth fragments, he tried to regain his composure. Why is it always time for side-splitting laughter when Doc gets kicked, gored, stepped on or otherwise mutilated by some uncouth ruffian of a cow?

When we finished the calves and headed for the well to wash up, he surprised me by stating between stifled giggles, "Any feller who gits stomped that bad and still finishes the job can't be such a bad vet."

Getting knocked down and stomped by an enraged yearling is probably not good stallside manner, and I don't ordinarily recommend it to young veterinarians. However, in the above incident, that particular dairyman became a good client of mine from that day on.

Good stallside manner is not getting riled when clients come into the animal clinic and declare, "Why, y'all are just as busy as real doctors." Then they say, "Why didn't you just become a R.D. (real doctor)?"

I've always wanted to get right up in their left ear and holler, " 'Cause I despise people!!"

Obviously, that's not true. I believe that veterinarians must like and enjoy people, as well as their animals, to be a good practitioner. And that's the basis for good stallside manner.

7

The old barn

I HAD seen the old barn many times in passing and even had seen the shorthorn-looking cows and yearlings in the lot or standing under the added-on lean-to out of the rain. But I never had been invited there to render my services as an animal doctor until now.

The delapidated structure was located right next to the gravel road and was set at an odd angle so that the rear corner of the lean-to was less than three feet from the fence guarding the road. The eave actually hung out over the edge of the ditch. Also, the thing was leaning badly.

I began to notice, as I passed there in late afternoon, that there were people inside the barn milking the few cows by hand and probably hoping the barn wouldn't fall over before they finished.

The milk can always was sitting just outside where the door used to be before it fell off. I noticed that they were very careful to send only clean milk to the cheese plant since they always had a clean fertilizer sack stretched over the strainer, in order to filter out all the impurities.

That morning the grandmother, Mrs. Turner, had called requesting assistance.

"Mr. McCormack," she said seriously, "we've got a cow that's done gone plum crazy. I believe that a mad dog must've bit 'er!"

"How's she acting, Mrs. Turner?" I asked.

"Oh, she's actin' real nervous. She's been doin' that pert near all mornin.' Reckin she's got the hydrophobie?"

"Well, she could have. We do see it every now and then. When did she freshen?"

"She came in 'bout a month ago, and she was given' a Borden bucket full twice a day till this here happened," she lamented. "We won't be here today, but the cow will be

24

under the shed on the side of the barn when you get here."

I always have liked treating cows with nervous acetonemia because they respond so quickly to intravenous
glucose. I was sure that this cow was suffering from this
mysterious metabolic malady.

Physiologists have a field day when lecturing on acetonemia, or ketosis, as some call it. These experts go into
great and boring detail when trying to explain Kreb's Cycle and how the complex metabolic pathways operate in
order to keep blood glucose levels at proper levels.

Simply put, though, cows with ketosis don't get enough
energy, so they convert too much of their body fat to glucose. A side effect of this is the accumulation of the poten-
tially toxic ketone bodies. Why some cows go "loco" when
they get acetonemia and others don't is unknown, but it
surely must have something to do with the blood level of
those ketone bodies and their "addling" effect upon the
brain.

When I stopped at the barnyard gate, I spied the old
black Jersey cow under the lean-to rhythmically licking
the side of the corncrib. It was as if she had a natural crav-
ing for old oak boards.

As I drew closer to the old barn, I began to smell the unmistakable sweet oniony odor of a ketotic cow's breath. I
just knew then that she was going to be "healed" in minutes few!

Chaos commenced . . .

She paid no attention to me until I moved to catch her
with my rope. The instant I had it secured around her
neck, chaos commenced. She crashed into the side of the
crib, bellowed wildly and started bucking and leaping
around under the shed as if she had been converted instantly into a vicious, stiff-legged rodeo bull.

I was shocked and unprepared for this sudden and violent surge of activity. As the berserk bovine bandied and
ricocheted against the fragile barn walls and artistically
created long and deep scars in the soft dirt floor with her
hooves, I quickly scanned the cramped premises for a suit-
able anchor post. There was none. However, the situation
demanded that my end of the jerking rope be secured immediately to something more substantial and less movable

than my left forearm, so I quickly selected a support post that only was semirotten and looped the rope around it.

It was a mistake. This fact became evident about five seconds later as the irritated cow kept up her onslaught on the shabby structure. She continued to bellow, with tongue lolling out, and her breathing was becoming raspy and loud as she pulled against the support beam with all her strength.

Suddenly, the post buckled in the middle and the building started to creak and groan. The next thing I knew there was a popping crash, and I was left holding a "clothes-lined" lariat with an insane cow on the other end. In the middle was an old cedar post twirling around the rope like a majorette's baton. Beams began to pop and gnarly sheets of tin began to rain down on the two panicky occupants of the barn. The noise of falling lumber and timbers was deafening for what seemed to be a couple of minutes but, in reality, was only about three seconds.

Presently I found myself lying on my back, with boards, tin and flakes of hay stacked randomly on top of me. Dust was billowing everywhere.

I realized that the cow was nowhere to be seen, but I did hear a strange licking sound coming from the vicinity of the tractor. At least she had escaped the predicament that had befallen me and was back trying to eat the flywheel off the John Deere.

"Why do I get myself in these messes?" I recall saying to myself. All my veterinarin friends never had these troubles, or so they said. They could wear suits or white coveralls in their practices and never get them dirty! But I always was getting into these fixes!

I began thrashing around, knocking tin and planks aside with my number eleven, four-buckle overshoes. Eventually, I was able to move rafters over to one side enough so that I could crawl to safety.

I was trying to brush the dirt off my pants when the mailman, whom we called "Goat," stopped and peered out his car window.

"Doc, did you do that?" he asked, curiously, as he peered at the massive pile of kindling.

"Go on, Goat," I ordered, "just deliver yo' cards and letters. Can't you see I'm up to my neck in problems?"

He drove off in a huff.

The cow still had my rope around her neck, and she was now eating and licking on the tractor's right rear tire. I slipped up the rope and quickly looped it around the drawbar. Let's see if she could pull the tractor off!

In spite of her twisting, flipping and throwing herself on the ground, I finally got her injected with dextrose. When I released the rope, she went to the trough, drank water and then headed for the hay rack. She was eating with gusto when I realized that a strong wind was blowing out of the southwest. Dust was being kicked up, tin was rattling and drops of rain were piercing my skin.

On the way home I tried to come up with a diplomatic way of telling Mrs. Turner that I accidentally had razed her barn. I sure hoped she wouldn't sue! 'Course, since the cow had made such a dramatic recovery, maybe she would be lenient with me.

The storm was getting worse now and even hail began to fall. I was glad that I had finished with the Turner cow and catastrophe before this bad weather arrived.

Late that afternoon my wife called me on the two-way.

"Mrs. Turner was just on the phone, and she was pretty excited," she said.

"Well, uh, uh, what did she say? I asked.

"Oh, she said that the cow you treated this morning was completely well."

"What else did she say?" I asked.

"Well, she said that you were a great doctor, and she was most appreciative. That was her best cow."

"Is that all?"

"They had some excitement with their barn," she continued. "Seems they must've had a tornado touch down there during that bad cloud today, and it tore their barn down. She said that it was a miracle that the cow wasn't killed since she stayed under that shed most of the time. Wasn't that luck?"

"Yep," I smiled. "We were *all* very, very lucky today!"

If Goat, the mailman, ever realized that he saw the barn collapse *before* the tornado, he never did say so . . .

27

8

Always wave at the police

MOST veterinarians, who are busy livestock practitioners, usually are fast drivers. Somehow we always are late
for our next appointment or we have that emergency that
needs attention. This habit seems to put us in frequent contact with the law.

"Always wave at t' police!" advised Sam Pete Smith,
family friend and amateur career-development counselor.
Sam flunked out of the first grade before Thanksgiving but
probably had more common sense than all the Washington, D.C. residents combined. We called his utterances and
pronouncements "Sam's Sayings." When I finally learned
that I really didn't know everything, I clamped my lips
shut and listened intently whenever Sam spoke.

Sam believed that you should develop a good rapport
with motoring law types, that the lines of communication
between regular folks and the sheriff's office should be
open, and that meaningful dialogue with state troopers
should be established. Actually, Sam just believed in trying to get along with others, especially if those others wore
a badge and other items that resembled Army or Navy
surplus on their wide leather belts.

Sam even knew the names of all the area game wardens
and was extra nice to the federal boys, since they had more
authority and knew less about normal farming practices.
That came in handy when trying to explain how those dove
fields got all that extra wheat on them.

So, when I went into practice, I took Sam's advice. I
learned who all the law types were, their names, the
names of their dogs, who their friends were and where
they hung out to drink coffee. When I would come up on a
wreck on the highway, I'd radio in to my office and have
them call the proper authority. When I met those official

cars on the highway, I'd blink my lights and wave big, like Porter Waggoner, the country music star, does at the end of his TV dividends.

One day, for example, I was flying down the highway, trying to get to an Angus heifer in labor, when a deputy sheriff started his siren behind me.

"Doc, where you goin' in such a hurry, Boy?" he asked from behind those jumbo sunglasses when he finally caught up.

"Thank goodness you came along, depitty," I said in a relieved voice. "Could yo' please escort me quickly up to Commissioner Clark's farm? His best heifer is in severe labor!"

"Uh, sure, sure, Doc," he stammered. "Just follow me!"

Just being polite to the nice officer got me off the hook. Of course, using the word "commissioner" didn't hurt anything either, since the commissioners control the county money.

Not many folks have had state troopers stop them and then later apologize. One evening my wife, Jan, and I had been out to dinner and a movie. I had been required to wear a suit and tie and my Sunday slippers. When I scratched off in Jan's new white station wagon from a four-way stop, a parked trooper tore out after me and flagged me to a stop. He looked us over and then warned me about jack rabbit starts.

The next morning he stopped by the clinic and came in to see me while I was trimming a sleeping Great Dane's ears.

"Doc, I'm sorry 'bout last night," he apologized. "I thought you were a drunk when you tore out from that intersection."

"Aw, that's plum awright, **officer**. You were just doing your usual fine and alert job!"

"The problem was that I didn't recognize you without your sleeveless coveralls and rubber boots," he said.

All that waving, grinning and light blinking had paid off again!

Out-of-state law types aren't too impressed with unknown vets. Recently, when my students and I were working in another state, a big, burly patrolman stopped me for speeding.

"But officer, we're on our way up to Mr. Butler's place to do some real important animal health work!" I pleaded.

"Oh, you're going up to the Butler's, eh? Good folks, good folks — lemme see them driver's license again. Yep, Mrs. Butler fixes the best coconut cake in the state. I'll have to keep yo' license till you pay this fine — everybody loves those people!"

"Yes sir, they're some of my favorite people," I said pleadingly, "and I'd sure hate for some of those little calves to die on account of us runnin' late."

"Aw, I know it. I hope the little boogers ain't too sick — just mail that fine in before the 25th, Hon, and I spec' there won't be no trouble — give the Butlers my best regards when you get there!"

Meanwhile, the students were hiding inside the van, giggling at my unfortunate fate and trying to take a picture of me with my head bowed, face flushed, and lower lip bit. I have been hearing about this incident ever since.

The strangest incident occurred in my own driveway several months ago. It was at midnight after an alumni gathering and class reunion. One of my poultry veterinarian buddies called and had the usual heifer in labor and asked for my help. He thought she was trying to deliver a two-headed calf.

I quietly got out of bed without waking my wife, then sleepily walked outside and started searching all around the house for my lariat and halter. With a big flashlight, I searched under the deck, on the front porch, and around behind the house, all the time moving junk around and showering the premises with generous beams of light. Finally I found an old half-rotten plowline, got into the truck, and sleepily drove out the driveway.

As I started to ease onto the paved road, all of a sudden a county police car appeared like a flash from out of the field across the road and slid sideways to a stop, blocking my progress. Multiple blue lights were flashing, and the long fishing-pole radio antenna was whipping crazily at all angles as the stern-faced constable exited his car and blinded me with his Radio Shack flashlight.

"Get outta that car real slow like," he ordered from his hiding place behind the car door.

"Wha-what's this all about, Mr. Police?" I stammered.

"I seen you over there trying to rogue that chainsaw from behind that feller's house!" he said.

"Buddy, I live there!" I offered in disbelief.

"Sho' nuff?" he sneered. "Then lemme see some ID."

I shakily got out my billfold and handed him a Gulf credit card and Red Cross blood donor card. He examined them carefully.

"I'm sorry, sir," he apologized. "We've had so many break-ins round here, we're just watching things real close. What are you doing out so late?"

"Well, I'm just going over to help deliver a two-headed calf in a chicken house behind the golf course."

I should not have said it. It was too much for him to accept or believe. He jumped back about 10 feet, unsnapped his holster strap and drew his gun on me.

"O.K., Mister," he said as he steadied the thing with both hands. "Just git out of the car, put your hands on top, and spread eagle them legs!"

Have you ever tried to explain the facts about bovine obstetrics to someone whose only contact with cows has been through a half-day trip to the zoo when he was 6? He couldn't understand why someone would be out in the middle of the night fooling with cows.

Finally, I suggested that we go back to the house and my wife would clear up the matter.

"O.K.," he said, "get in the car and we'll see what she says."

When we arrived in the front of the house, he surprised me by ordering me to stay inside the car. He charged up the steps and rapped on the door while keeping an eye on a barking mutt.

My wife, Jan, finally came to the door, yawning and tying her bathrobe.

" 'Scuse me, Madam," said the lawman with hat in hand. "Is Mr. McCormack at home?"

"He sure is, officer," she said. "He's downstairs sound asleep."

I started beating on the window and trying to get out. Did you know that the rear doors of police cars have no handles?

"Jan, it's me, it's me!" I yelled frantically. "Tell the policeman that it's me!"

With a stunned look on her face, she assured the officer that I was indeed a resident of the house and that if I had said that I was going to deliver a two-headed calf, that was correct. After an apology, the officer left. I was glad to know that the law was looking out after us. The calf delivery was routine — no two-headed fetus!

In spite of some of my experiences with law enforcement officers, I know of no group of people who are so grossly underpaid, overcriticized or are in more constant danger. I respect them and my hat is off to them.

9

The milk can snatcher

E-52. That was the red number painted on the side of all our milk cans. E route, and I reckon we were the 52nd milk pick-up on that route. The Jersey milk was picked up at the end of the driveway twice a day in summer and once a day in the winter and hauled to Mr. Jones' cheese plant in Ardmore, Tenn.

One of my most detested chores was to wheelbarrow the milk to the pick-up point at the driveway's end. Depending upon the milk flow, we'd usually have one to two cans of milk to send. The wheelbarrow that we had was designed to be pushed by big, heavy-muscled, grown adult types, not a bare-footed kid who barely could reach the handles.

Often I'd wait for the milk truck just to marvel at the can snatcher at work. He just had to be the strongest guy around, the way he tossed those full cans of milk around. After the milk truck had picked up the full cans and left the empties, I'd pick them up and wheel them back to the barn.

The return trip with the empties wasn't all that bad, except it was uphill. So I'd work up a pretty rapid heartbeat just moving milk cans.

Now the interesting part of this everyday affair was the milk hauling duo, the driver and can snatcher, and their milk pick-up and can drop-off techniques. The can snatcher (hereafter designated as CS) was the most interesting part of this team.

People who snatched cans usually were "cool" guys. They were well-muscled, football-player types who were well-tanned and went shirtless or at least had their shirt sleeves whacked off at the shoulders. They drove mufflerless Model A Ford roadsters mounted on 6:00 x 16 tires, quit school in the 10th grade, hung around the pool hall and were strong as oxen. They had names like Buck, Thrillkill or Scarface. Girls liked them.

The CS rode in the back of the covered milk truck and it was his simple duty to drop off the empty cans and pick up the full ones. The truck body had a side-to-side alleyway with open doors on each side, just above the dual wheels.

The CS carried out his job using one of two basic techniques. The E route technique called for the CS to crouch in the doorway, with the handles of the empties in both hands. When the milk pick-up point was approached, he suddenly sprung into action. He gently tossed the empties out with a twirling action, so they would land and remain upright at a point just adjacent to the full cans.

A second after the empties were airborne, he would hurl himself out of the doorway and, if his timing was correct and proper, would touch down just on the off side of the cans to be picked up. He then would vigorously attach himself to the handles of a full can and heave it, with a grunt, into the open door of the truck. The same process was repeated on the other full can(s).

He then signaled to the driver, by a whistle or yell, that his mission had been accomplished. Then quickly he stepped lightly on the turning axle hub and pulled himself back into the truck to arrange his newly acquired cans in their correct position. All this took place in a matter of a few seconds, and the driver never stopped the truck. He just slowed down some.

The B route technique came about after so many producers complained about dented cans. It was introduced after World War II by a discharged and halfway-addled paratrooper. In this technique, the CS leaped from the truck like a bullfrog, with empties in hands. He supposedly landed adjacent to the full cans and then loaded them in the same fashion as before. This supposedly led to increased longevity of cans, but, unfortunately, it led to decreased longevity of the CS. Toes, ankles and elbows were especially vulnerable.

Mistakes commonly made by neophyte or careless CS's included spilling of milk, unnecessarily rough treatment of cans, tossing full cans up into the truck with too much vigor and having them roll out the other side, losing cans, throwing cans too far out from the pick-up zone and putting the wrong cans out. Other prospective CS's washed out because they took too long, constantly smashed their toes under cans or were left behind by a daydreaming driver when they couldn't get back into the truck quickly enough.

The driver had to be skillful in his own right. He had to be able to gear down the GMC and go slow enough at the critical phase to coordinate his efforts with those of the CS. Brakes were used sparingly. Drivers had names like Foot Crusher, Leadfoot, Smiling Jack, or Cowboy.

The hardest part about being a driver was that frequently he had to both drive and snatch cans, if the regular CS and substitute CS were indisposed. On those days you didn't want to be around him, since he could be heard mumbling in unknown tongues. For some strange reason, bad headaches, broken jaws, knife wounds and other similar type of traumatic injuries plagued the CS fraternity and these injuries often led to frequent absenteeism.

At one time, I really wanted to become a can snatcher on B route but Dad wouldn't let me quit school in the 10th grade to do so.

"Thanks, Dad!"

10

Lige whispered in her ear

DOC, I need you to come over here and see 'bout a cow that's down,'' the person on the other end of the buzzing line declared.

It was Clay Boozer, a part-time cattleman, pulpwood dealer and dedicated football fan. He was fanatic about the Alabama Crimson Tide and the late Coach Bear Bryant. Clay was a "good feller," his neighbors all said, but his constant carrying on about Alabama football tested my patience, as well as that of many others.

I secured a little history about the cow and then promised Clay I'd be there within a couple of hours, since I had to check in on a colicky mule along the way.

Downer cows that have been unable to rise for several days are some of the most dreaded calls.

Years ago, downer cows usually meant milk fever, and they hopped right up with much enthusiasm after receiving a warm jug of calcium. Nowadays, it seems that downer cows frequently are suffering from complex metabolic problems, and they do not respond well to the usual therapy.

Clay's cow was suffering from chronic malnutrition. This sounds a little better than "starvation." Different people respond differently to a diagnostic suggestion. Over the years, a few farmers have challenged me to fist fights when I have diagnosed starvation too quickly. I have learned that, in some cases, it is better to diplomatically call the condition "high trough disease," or "internal energy deficiency complex," or "abomasal filling defect."

The cow in question had found the deepest part of the woods, as most do when in trouble, to claim as her hospital ward.

Upon arrival at cowside, I found that the old Hereford-

36

Jersey cross was being attended by Clay's main hand, an elderly man named Lige. Lige truly was ancient, and the best description of him would be to call him a "throwback." He was kind of a veterinarian, too, but his practice methods were suspect. I had followed him on several occasions, and I knew that he treated mostly for "holler tail," "holler horn," and "the Murrah." My own reputation in the community had been summed up pretty well by another farmer at the store one day.

Get Lige for "Murrah" . . .

"Doc's pretty good at calvings, prolapses and herd work," he bragged, "but he ain't worth a dern on the Murrah."

I still don't know what "The Murrah" is, but I let on like I did.

"What do you reckon's wrong with this old cow, Lige?" I asked diplomatically, as I started at her rear parts and worked forward with my examination.

"I reckon she's got the holler tail, suh," he said, apologetically, as I seized her by the nose, pulled down her lower lip and checked her teeth. Her incisors were gone, except for nubs that were worn down flush with the gumline.

"How old do you think she is, Clay?" I asked, just to see what he'd say.

"Aw, let's see, Doc," he allowed, as he thought. "I think I got her at the sale barn the year that Alabama played Tulane a night game in Mobile at Ladd Stadium, and she was a yearling at the time. So I guess she's 10."

"Look at those teeth, Clay! She's old enough to vote!" I exclaimed. "And look at her condition; she's so thin there's nothing here but skin and bones. Plus she's got a big calf in her. She hasn't got a chance!"

"But, Doc, I remember one night you came over to Miss Molly's place over here to an old Jersey milk cow that was down. You gave her a shot, and she jumped right up."

"Clay, that was milk fever, not starvation, and it won't work quite that easy," I said.

"Lige wanted to split her tail and put salt and pepper in it for the holler tail, but I told him yo' medicine was better," Clay allowed.

"Well, let me tell you this!" I declared. "I guarantee

that splitting her tail and putting stuff in it is not gonna get her up!"

"O.K. Clay, here's what we'll do," I said. "We'll give her a bunch of gluclose and I.V. fluids, then some vitamin injections. If we don't make a first down with that game plan, then we'll pass a stomach tube and pump gruel and grits into her. If we don't gain yardage with that, then we'll put the hip lift on her and pick her up twice a day. If we haven't scored by then, we'll punt and you can fire the coach. Does that sound like a good plan?"

"I believe we ought to split her tail . . ."

"We're not going to do that," I yelled. "Just get that notion out of your head!"

The treatment was carried out, and I left medication there for them to give. Clay called every other night to report on her progress or the lack of it. He always suggested that we consider allowing Lige to perform tail surgery.

Nursing downers becomes very frustrating, especially when the cow loses her spirit and gives up. Clay gave up one Sunday afternoon after about four weeks.

"Doc, can you come over here and put this old cow out of her misery?" he requested. "I just can't keep on doctorin' her."

"Why sure, Clay, but why don't you just use that deer rifle?"

"I just can't do it, Doc. You come on and give her one of them sleepin' shots."

"Doc, you are not gonna like this," he continued, "but Lige kept on after me about splittin' that cow's tail, so I let him go on down there a while ago and do it."

"Yeah, you're right," I said haughtily, "I don't like it. But it's your cow, and you can do what you want with her."

On the way to the woods, I said, "Clay, you've just got to realize that nothing, and I mean absolutely nothing, could have been done to save that cow. She was a goner from the start. Don't second guess our treatment."

Finally, we completed our rough passage through the rocky pasture and started slowly down the logging trail to where our doomed patient was located.

Suddenly, Clay sprung to the edge of the passenger seat, quickly wiped off the inside of the windshield and blinked his eyes.

"Doc, do you see what I see coming up the trail, or am I seeing a 'haint'?" he stammered.

As I strained to look down the trail through the bushes and briars, I could make out a briskly moving figure. As we both stared, open-mouthed, the old cow that was down and knocking at death's door only a few hours before, came marching up the logging trail. She reminded me of an old crippled soldier, proudly marching during a Veteran's Day parade. I could almost hear the band playing the Marine's Hymn as she trudged up the hill and paused briefly in front of my truck as if it were a reviewing stand. I thought for a moment that she was going to salute. Instead, with eyes blinking, she just stared at us.

With a switch of her bandaged tail, she stomped by the truck, made her way out into the pasture and began sampling some of the young clover.

It hit Clay and me at the same instant. The bandaged tail! That meant that Lige had done it! We both turned back towards the trail just in time to see Lige emerge from the woods. He was grinning from ear to ear and was carrying a half-pound box of Watkins black pepper in one hand and a box of Morton's salt in the other. The remnants of an old sheet dangled from his rear pocket.

What Lige had done was to make a liberal incision with his pocket knife just above the tail switch at the open space where the bones play out. He had poured copious amounts of pepper and salt into the open incision and then wrapped the wound with strips of an old sheet. A bow knot adorned the finished product.

"Lige, what made her get up?" I asked, trying to mask the shock that was showing on my face.

"Well, suh," he drawled, "ah jus' done her tail lack always and then urged her to git up. She didn't so ah whispered in her ear."

"What did you tell her, Lige?" Clay asked impatiently.

"Ah tole her that this was Mr. Coach Bear Bryant speakin' and that she was s'posed to rise an' walk. Then she slowly got to her feet and tried to run off."

"Why'd you say that?" I asked.

"Well, I used to hear Mr. Clay all time talkin' so much 'bout Mr. Coach Bryant and how he could walk on water and keep it from rainin' on ball-game day. So I figured that he could easy git an ole cow up off the groun'.''

I still don't understand the mechanism involved in getting that old cow up. I'm not sure that I want to know. What I did learn from that incident was that I never should guarantee what treatment won't work.

11

"Go to preachin' every Sunday"

I WAS all robed out and sitting in the choir loft when the phone rang back in the office of the small church. I figured that it probably was for me. It rang a second time, but still I sat motionless in the cane-bottomed and hard-backed chair. Several of my choirmates were beginning to tap their feet nervously, twist their heads and peer anxiously in my general direction.

If the preacher was bothered by the jingling of the phone, he didn't let it show. Instead, he just kept on pounding the pulpit and letting the congregation know in no uncertain terms that Sunday golf and everyday carousing were going to be the ruination of all mankind.

On the third ring, J. B. Malone, the head usher, arose quietly from the same pew that he had occupied regularly for the past 74 years or more and tried to tiptoe out over the creaking wooden floor towards the back door. He glared up at me with lips pursed as he shuffled past the choir. I knew exactly what he was thinking.

"Dang yo' time, Doc! This is the third Sunday in a row that somebody's called in heah interruptin' this here service with a sick cow or somethin'."

Now I could hear J. B. conversing loudly with the calling party. J. B. always hollered over the phone since he figured that the person on the other end was a long way off.

"Just a minute," he bellowed. "I'll see if I can find 'im."

He knew very well where I was sitting, but the cranky rascal had to be difficult about it.

When he creaked open the door and sneeringly nodded his head in my direction, I already was in motion, trying to stand up and ease out as unobtrusively as possible. Naturally, all eyes were on the guy slipping out the back door. All eyes except the preacher's, since he still was busy chewing everybody out. Now he was getting into card playing and folks that worked on Sunday. Maybe he didn't mean veterinarians.

As I headed to the phone, my mind flashed back to what Sam Pete Smith had advised.

"Try to make it to preachin' every Sunday morning," the wise and revered sage often lectured. And since his common sense and wisdom were legendary, I usually tried to follow his advice.

Getting to preaching isn't always easy for animal doctors and owners of livestock. Cows often pick very inopportune times to get sick or give birth to their young.

That morning at 10:30 for instance, I had roped a skittish Holstein heifer in a farm pond, dragged her out, delivered her calf, cleaned up and changed clothes and still made it to church only 10 minutes late. 'Course I had to pull on my choir robe quickly and crawl on my stomach from the side door into the choir loft while the preacher was praying. When he finally said "Amen," I was sitting in a chair like all the others, as if getting to church had been just a leisurely morning accomplishment and not the time-defying act it really was.

I always was getting called out of civic meetings, too! Just a couple of weeks ago, I had been conducting a town utilities board meeting when suddenly someone rapped urgently on the closed door.

"Come on in," I shouted, since I figured it was the town's newspaper editor.

When the door flew open, in walked a frantic-looking, middle-aged lady with blue hair and her meek, head-bowed husband. She was wringing her hands. He was playing with his hat.

"Oh, Mr. McCormack, I'm so glad I've found you," she sobbed. "I've just had a horrible thing to happen!" She had a paper sack under her arm.

"Well, just settle down," I said soothingly as I tried to usher the two back outside. The board members were somewhat taken aback by this unusual event.

"Oh, my husband slammed the car door on little Poochie's tail and amputated it!" she screamed, emphasizing "amputated."

With this news, my colleagues sprung to their feet and

42

inched forward to the door, trying to hear more about the tragic event.

"Well, did you bring the dog?" I asked.

"No," she replied, "but I've brought his tail. Here it is in this grocery sack." She reached in and brought out a three-quarter-inch piece of dog tail.

Most of my fellow board members were not exactly companion animal enthusiasts, so they couldn't put themselves in the poor lady's shoes. Instead, they all erupted into cheek-popping guffawing when the amputated tail was retrieved from the sack for viewing. I wanted to choke every last one of them!

I promised to go straight to the clinic after the meeting if they could find the "tail-tipless" dog. I tried to continue with the important town meeting, but we finally had to adjourn because of the multitude of jokes and laughing that was interfering with the city's business.

This Sunday morning, as I picked up the phone, I wondered what type of serious emergency it would be, probably a prolapsed uterus, colicky mare or bloated steer; or perhaps it was a poodle hit by a reckless driver headed to the lake or a child's pony bleeding to death.

"Hello, this is Dr. McCormack," I said, real concerned-like. "May I help you?"

"Hey, Doc, you got any of them big red worm pills for dogs?" a laid-back voice inquired. "I got this here coon dog that's been ailin' all week an' I figure he needs a good wormin'."

"Who is this?" I asked curtly. I could feel my face burning and the hair standing up on the back of my neck.

"This is Buck, Doc," he said in a surprised tone. There were only about 2,000 "Bucks" in my practice vicinity. "How 'bout them pills?"

"Tell you what, Buck," I said nicely, "let me check my supply, and I'll call you back next week!" Then, with teeth gritted and eyes narrowed, I gently laid the phone back into its cradle, just in time to rush back to the choir and help sing the last two verses of "Love Lifted Me!"

Going to preaching doesn't make a better or more skillful person out of any of us, but it may make us better able to tolerate the "Bucks" of this world.

12

"Aw, Doc, we'll be through by 7"

VETERINARIANS and dairymen probably hold the world's record for being late to appointments, meetings and recitals.

"Better late than never," Dan Cabaniss said the other night as he came stomping and tracking mud into the dairy meeting about 8:30 p.m. Farmers usually pay little notice if someone else comes in late since it is such a common occurrence. Regular civilian folks can't understand it.

"Doc, I've got a bunch of calves that need to be vaccinated, castrated and implanted," explained Sonny Brewer one April evening.

"Well, Sir, you sure called the right place," I joked. "We're running a special on that this week!"

"Good, good!" he allowed. "I'll have 'em penned and ready to go after work Tuesday afternoon. I'll be ready about 6."

"Uh, wait a minute Sonny," I said, hesitating, "I think my little girl has a piano recital that night about 7:30."

"Aw, we'll be through by 7, Doc," he said convincingly. "You know it won't take long to work those 30 or so calves."

I knew it was a mistake when I agreed, but I did it anyway. Sonny did have a good corral and squeeze chute and, if all went well, it wouldn't take long. Of course, if he had trouble getting them penned, or if one fool calf got turned around in the alleyway or upside down in the squeeze, then I'd be held up and would be late again. But, if I didn't get them done on Tuesday, it would be way into next week before I could get to it. By then he either would have done it himself, gotten someone else or have forgotten the whole thing.

"Daddy, don't forget my piano recital tomorrow night,"

said my little Lisa as she hugged me goodnight on Monday. "I've been practicing real hard on my solo just so it will be perfect for you."

"Don't you worry, Lisa Bug, I'll be right there," I said as I knocked on wood. "I may not be there right at 7:30, but I'll be there for your part. I'll probably be standing in the back by the door."

Tuesday went real well. I was on time everywhere I went. The cattle all behaved unusually well, and I caught a minimum of emergencies. I just felt like all was going according to plan so that I could make Lisa's recital.

It was 5:55 when I pulled up in front of Sonny's corral. His truck was there, but I could see no sign of him or the calves. Uh oh! I knew this was going to happen.

As I began to stomp, spit and nervously twiddle the implants in my pocket, I heard Sonny yell.

"Yo! Yo! Yo!" he was saying to the beasts. Then I could see him coming over the hill with a coffee can full of range cubes under his right arm. He was teasing the calves by offering them an occasional cube while walking slowly toward the catch pen. He would walk a few steps, then stop and exchange pleasantries with random calves. This went on for several minutes. My watch said 6:10. I couldn't stand it any longer!

"Sonny, please hurry up!" I pleaded diplomatically, "I ain't got all night!"

"Shhh! Doc," he indicated by putting his finger to his lips.

I just sat down on the ground beside the truck on the side away from the corral fence and fumed. I could hear him talking and getting closer to the pen. It was 6:20.

"Whoap, whoap!" I heard Sonny say, just as he got to the gate. At that moment, I heard a shuffling, earth-gouging commotion and the sounds of hot bovine flesh bumping into creosoted two by tens. The gate slammed shut loudly amidst the chaos and I immediately detected the depressing sound of numerous cloven hooves slowly fading away.

"Got half of em, Doc!" Sonny chirped proudly. "It won't take but 10 minutes more to get the others back up. They're just a little nervous with your new white truck parked there. Is that a four-wheel drive or what, Doc? Sure is nice, got that nice telephone body and all . . ."

"Sonny, I'll swear!" I screeched, "I'm in a big hurry, Man! I don't have time to talk trucks. Get those wild calves in here so I can get through!" My watch said 6:23.

Suddenly, as if a higher power had decided to assist, the calves that had escaped started loping back toward the pen.

"Open the gate! Open the gate!" I whispered loudly.

While keeping an eye on the trapped group, Sonny eased open the gate, and within minutes the other calves had, for some strange reason, walked into the pen. To this day, I do not understand why.

"Fill the alleyway full, Sonny," I ordered. "I'll just walk down the side, vaccinate all of them and implant the bulls. Then we'll catch the bulls' heads."

I was carrying my syringe and implant gun in makeshift holsters strapped to my side so I could make quick work of vaccinating.

As I jabbed the first bellowing patient, my watch read 6:35. I'd have to work fast! When I finished vaccinating the first group, I jumped in amongst the beasts and started pushing the heifers out as Sonny opened and closed the headgate. As I castrated the last bull, my watch read 7:22.

"Sonny, I'm gone," I yelled as I streaked for the truck. "I'd help you clean up and all, but I'm already late!"

"Well, I wanted you to look at the knot on that horse's leg, Doc," he drawled slowly, "but I reckon we can do that another night. That dog needs wormin', too, and a rabies shot . . ."

As I cranked the truck and roared away, I still could see Sonny's lips moving, and I knew that he still was unconcerned about time and was thinking up more for me to do.

Have you ever tried to change from dirty coveralls to clean clothes while driving? It's not easy, but I did it that night as the truck rocketed towards the schoolhouse. I drove right up to the auditorium, parked right in everyone's way, bolted up the steps four at a time and hit the door just as the audience was applauding Molly Jackson's solo.

Lisa was next. As she marched pertly across the stage toward the piano, I thought to myself:

"Isn't she the prettiest little girl anyone has ever seen?" Her hair was back in a pony tail, and she was wearing a pretty, fluffy little yellow dress and those funny little shoes with a strap over the top. Her mother always fixed her up so pretty.

As she sat down on the bench, adjusted it and began to play with much concentration and confidence, I suddenly was filled with pride and emotion. This is what life is all about! I was glad that it was dark in the back of the auditorium so that none of my friends could see my glassy eyes. I also realized how nervous I had been about her first public piano performance. There was no way that she could have been as nervous as her father.

When she finished, I could see my wife, Jan, leading the hand clapping. Lisa stood, curtsied and left the stage briskly. But just before she went behind the curtain she looked toward the door where I was standing and waved discreetly. She knew I was there!

When the recital ended, Lisa was the first one down the steps. She made a beeline to me.

"How did I do, Daddy?" she asked excitedly.

"Aw, you did just great, Honey," I replied. "I'm proud of you for practicing so hard and doing such a good job."

Many people who work late or are on call surely do miss one of life's greatest pleasures when they don't see their children in plays, recitals, ball games and the like. I know; I've missed way too many.

13

Dairy meetings . . . I love 'em

I JUST love going to dairy and cattlemen's meetings! In my opinion, they are another one of life's numerous pleasures. Usually I'm in attendance because the county agent, who frequently is the program chairman, meeting-place securer, cook and other arrangement-maker, has invited me. In order to pay for my supper, they generally require that I put on a slide show and discussion on health problems in cattle.

Naturally, though, the highlight of the session is always the breaking of the bread. Sometimes it will be a regular meal in the town cafe's small meeting room where the Rotarians and Lions meet, or it may be hamburgers grilled out behind the schoolhouse. If luck is with the group, it may be a nice steak that is being paid for by a feed and supply company, the bank or another loan agency. My favorite meal, though, is the covered dish supper or lunch. Others call this a potluck dinner.

Several years ago a number of us extension-service-types were putting on an all-day mastitis prevention seminar in a tiny community center building in north Georgia. As usual, the veterinarian's portion came at 11 a.m., right before lunch. I think the folks who set these programs up always put the vet on right before lunch so that, after he gets through talking about gangrenous mastitis, Staph mastitis and other appetite-depressing topics, the attendees will be sort of semi-nauseated and won't eat much.

Signs of late lunchitis . . .

While I was doing my part, I kept hearing a dish-rattling commotion outside in the approximate vicinity of where dinner-on-the-grounds usually was served. I couldn't see out the windows, though, since they were covered with dark curtains. About 12:15, I noticed the audience getting restless, as they commenced shuffling their feet, looking and listening at their watches, making rubbing motions on their stomachs and generally not paying any attention to what I was saying. I recognized those classic signs of late lunchitis, and, thus, quickly brought my lecture to an end.

"If there aren't any questions or comments, then we'll stand adjourned," I announced.

Immediately, some big, old half-grown boys hit the side door. They acted like two cows trying to exit the stall door simultaneously, the way they kind of got jammed and hung there by their hips, pushing and shoving, for a few seconds. They knew dinner was awaitin'!

When the rest of us finally walked outside, squinting in the bright sunshine, I saw a table about 30 feet long, piled high with numerous types of home-cooked victuals. There was fried chicken, collard greens, all kinds of peas, and pimento cheese sandwiches with the crusts cut off. I could see dish after dish of macaroni and cheese, sweet potatoes, corn on the cob, and all sorts of salads.

Several apron-wearing women were pacing back and forth behind the swaying-in-the-middle table like marching sentries, occasionally dispatching an unwelcome fly with an expert wave of a folded-up newspaper.

"Merciful heavens!" I declared, "I wondered what all the commotion was out here. Looks like a produce truck turned over on this table!"

Several of the ladies snickered proudly as they busied themselves rearranging the multitude of casseroles and desserts.

After "Amens" were said, plates were quickly piled high and then carried to the shade and comfort of a red oak tree, where the lovingly prepared eatables were consumed with much gusto.

The only problem with the scenario is that the number of return trips the hungry diners make to the table is directly proportional to the length of time those same participants will sleep during the afternoon "scientific" session.

In nearly every meeting that I attend, there is at least one "sleeper." A lot of us speakers are a little boring, I guess, so it is no wonder that little naps are taken while graphs, computer data and results of drug trials are being flashed on the screen. I know dairymen and other livestock owners are busy people who are up way before daylight and thus are ready for the waterbed right after supper. But it is a little distracting when the snores drown out my talking about calf hutches, ketosis or pinkeye.

Just the other night after supper, we had gotten into the slide show on a reproduction program when I heard this awful racket back in about the fifth row. As I droned on about cystic ovaries and metritis, I eased up closer to the audience to see what was making such a horrendous noise.

What I saw was one of my favorite dairyman clients, named Tommy, reared back in his chair, sound asleep. His head was flopped back over the church pew seat he was in, his mouth was open wide enough for a tonsillectomy and his arms kind of dangled on the seat. He had eaten so much steak and potatoes that he had unbuttoned his pants for easier breathing. His neighbors were looking around at him and stifling their snickering, while his slow 12 respirations per minute sounded like a growling bobcat trapped in the top of a persimmon tree.

After about three or four minutes of competing with him for the attention of the audience, a fly must have dove into his throat. All of a sudden he sprung upright in his seat, coughing and sputtering, his six-foot-four heavy frame mercilessly battering the wide-eyed sitters to either side.

"Huh! What, what, what is it?" he blurted out, still three-fourths asleep, as he looked around the room. "Is it milkin' time?"

Everybody had a big laugh at his expense, but I knew that I had lost the audience for good.

14

Beware of compliments from the boss

It WAS the first large animal call I had made in the new practice. The older veterinarian had saved it up just for me, by telling the owner just how smart and talented his newly hired young graduate was.

"He's just finished up and has learned all the latest surgical techniques," he had told the bull's owner. "Plus, he's a big ol' boy, good with a rope and stout as a mule. He's a whole lot better'n me at throwin' big ol' lame bulls down on the ground. I got this bad back you know."

Always be mighty suspicious of folks who brag on you and how good you are at doing some particular task. That means they are getting ready to pop it to you by "complimenting" you into doing the task. Bosses are real bad about this.

Also be suspicious of people who claim they have a bad back and can't do heavy work, like dehorning a few yearlings, but who have no difficulty at all playing golf or climbing up to their high level seats in the football stadium.

"Cyrus Boudreaux has this lil' ol' black bull with some swellings between his toes," the Bossman told me. "I want you to run out there and take 'em out for him. Mr. Boudreaux won't be there, he's on vacation."

"Yessir," I said doubtfully. "But I can't ever remember seeing corns in a little bull's feet before. Just how big is he?"

"Aw, just a yearlin', 'bout 1,800 pounds," he said with his mouth half covered up. "He's just a calf."

I don't know why folks do that to their colleagues. That's like these ads on TV that say they have a new truck down at the lot for $5,999, but when you get there it's $7,440, assuming you want wheels and a sun visor.

As I drove to the farm to surgically remove the corns

from the bull's feet, I was sort of nervous about the whole thing. How would Mr. Boudreaux react when he heard that a green, overgrown kid drove up and operated on his fine bull? I acted out every detail of the operation in my mind as I whizzed down by the bayou. I tried to think of how the bull might react at every point during the procedure, of every complication that could possibly arise. The more I thought about it, the more nervous I became. It was like a newly graduated professional singer getting ready to sing the national anthem at the packed Rose Bowl, who wasn't sure he or she knew the words.

As I rounded a bend in the road, I realized that there was truck after truck pulled over to the side of the road as if there had been a tragedy up ahead. As I eased slowly past the vehicles, I came up on a farmer walking briskly in the same direction.

"What happened?" I asked.

"Oh, Cyrus has got this big ol' mean bull down here, and the new cow doc thinks he's gonna cut them corns out from 'tween his toes," he said while laughing. "We're gonna see the rodeo!"

"Hey, you must be him!" he blurted out as the realization hit him that I was a stranger in a funny looking truck with one too many radio antennas.

"Yessir, I'm him," I stammered. "The bull's not all that mean, though, is he? My boss didn't mention a thing . . ."

"Is he mean? Is he mean? he screamed. "That bull tears out of that pasture over there just to attack red cars and trucks! He gored two dogs to death last Christmas! He broke Cokey Couvillon's leg in three places one night when Cokey came along here likkered up and got over in the bull lot by mistake!" he shouted.

I swallowed hard, and I'm sure my face blanched out. I could just see me having the shortest veterinary career in history.

"Aw, he's not really that bad, is he?" I asked in a dry throaty voice.

"Naw, he ain't mean, he's jus' a little darlin'," he sneered. "You'll find out soons as you step inside 'at barn over there, Mr. Hot Shot Vetnerry!"

I eased my truck past all the parked vehicles, through the open gate and right up to a sturdy, small barn. Every human eye, probably close to 40 pairs of them, was riveted on me, as I detrucked with fear, trepidation and absolutely no self-confidence remaining.

As I quickly surveyed the rough looking group of farmers, oil field workers and professional tobacco chewers, I noticed that not a single one of them was smiling. While I was wondering why, a series of strange but clearly identifiable noises began to come from inside the barn. The barn had no large door through which a load of hay could be driven. Instead, there were only a couple of small doors, just big enough to accommodate an adult bull or a chunky man, and a small window.

The noise coming from the door on the left was a typical bull bellow, followed by the sound of dirt and other stall debris and pebbles being hurled skyward to the tin roof by a viciously pawing hoof. Immediately following that, there was a bone-chilling snort which actually rattled the 1 by 8 cypress boards around the stall. Dust was flying out from under the bottom of the stall from all the snorting and bellowing that was going on. After about a 10 second seige of this, all would be silent for an equal amount of time, then the cycle would be repeated.

"Can any of y'all help me get him out of there into this lot?" I asked while retrieving nylon lariat, long casting ropes, tranquilizers and other paraphernalia from the truck.

Two cowboys stepped forward. One was about 6 foot 5 and the other one at least a foot shorter. They were certainly dressed for the part — chaps, cowboy boots and hats as big as umbrellas. I knew immediately that their names were "Mutt" and "Jeff."

After a short truckside conference, we trudged purposefully toward the barn. Our plan was to toss two strong lariats over the bull's neck from the small window that was in the back of the stall, then loop one of the ropes around a barn support post. The other rope would be passed through the barely open door and looped around a small tree just outside the door. Then I would inject him with a tranquilizer, and let him out the door before the drug had time to work.

It worked fairly well. It took several tosses to get the ropes over his head. Once caught, he choked himself down a couple of times due to his wild thrashing and pulling on the rope. While he was choked down the second time, I plunged the tranquilizer into his huge gluteal muscles and opened the door.

Upon seeing the daylight offered by the suddenly opened exit, the wild bull staggered to his corny feet and bolted toward freedom. I was trying to hang onto the lariat inside the barn, Jeff was holding tightly onto his rope on the outside, while Mutt was jumping around outside the door like a playful puppy, making faces and waving his hands at our patient.

Apparently, Mutt zagged when he should have zigged, and the next thing we knew, the snorting and charging bull was wearing Mutt over his face and between his stubby horns like an ill-fitting Halloween mask. Jeff and I were holding onto our ropes with all our strength, but the lariats were burning hot rings around the post and tree as the panic-stricken beast was quickly taking more and more rope out of our hands.

"He's loose!" shouted Jeff and I at the same instant, as the bellowing and bucking bull headed into the small tree-lined lot. Mutt, stuck between the bull's horns and unable to disengage himself from his dilemma, was yelling for help and trying not to fall off. The bull showed no signs of being lame at the moment.

The spectators were engaged in a variety of activities. Most of the professional fence sitters were cracking their sides with laughter and making no effort to save Mutt from severe injury. Others, who were less experienced in impromptu, unplanned rodeos, could be seen easing slowly away from the fence and heading towards the general direction of their vehicles. They were just sure that the rank bull was going to permanently disable old Mutt, then break through the rickety fence and start beating up on their trucks and cars.

Several of the more thoughtful of the group began scanning the ground for sticks, and then jumped into the corral in an effort to rescue the bull's latest victim. At the same time, Jeff and I were chasing the two around the lot, and one of us would occasionally grab at a snaking and jerking rope along the ground, only to have it snatched from our grasp just as we thought we had it.

Mutt's bull ride lasted less than 10 seconds, but with all the goings on, it seemed much longer, especially to he and I. The ride reached its conclusion when the bull suddenly stopped, but poor Mutt, who still had his hat firmly stuck on his head, kept traveling in midair until his backside made solid contact with a briar-infested corner of the lot.

Up to that point, only unmentionable type words had been exclaimed or uttered during the ride. Jeff was the first to speak a full sentence.

"Hoss, if I'd a'knowed y'wanted to ride, I'd a'brought muh mule!" he drawled amid stifled giggles and snickers from the remaining spectators.

"Y'all jus' shut up, heah!" Mutt shouted, as he picked himself up out of the briars and commenced picking sticks out of his clothes and scratched-up face. But he still had his 10-gallon hat tight on his head.

In the meantime, the exhausted bull was feeling the effects of the tranquilizer and was standing, with his head drooped low, over by the gate. I quietly walked over, picked up the end of one of the lariats, looped it around the gate post and tied it in a slip knot.

"Jeff, watch and don't let 'em joke while I go get my stuff," I said, as I climbed the fence and headed for the truck.

When I returned with all my surgical paraphernalia, the bull had decided to lay down and take a nap. All we had to do then was put our ropes on his extremities, stretch him out and tie him up tight.

While Mutt and Jeff haltered, tied and held down his head, I went to work scrubbing his back feet and anesthetizing the surgical site. Everything was going well now — I realized that I wasn't nervous anymore!

I have always enjoyed removing corns from cows' feet. Usually, the animal is quite lame beforehand, and they always do so much better after surgery. They just have to feel better after getting their feet fixed.

I had no trouble making the incisions, dissecting out the growths and putting in a couple of sutures. Then, as the bull snored lightly, I applied antibiotic powder and wrapped each foot with pretty white gauze and lots of 2-inch tape until the entire foot was covered in white. An injection of penicillin topped off the job. It was all over. All we had to do was remove all the restraining ropes, sit him up and get out of the way.

"Y'all move now," I ordered. "I don't know what this rascal's liable to do when he gets up!"

Mutt led the charge to the fence. He had seen enough bull for one day. Jeff was still trying to keep from laughing at Mutt, but couldn't help himself whenever he would look at his partner's torn-up clothes and scratched-up skin surfaces.

While everyone else watched from the safety of the fence, I eased up to the groggy bull, slapped him on the rump and jumped back out of range. The old bull arose very slowly, turned and looked at the audience and commenced grazing. No bellowing, no charging and no earth pawing. He just stood there chewing, looking like he had just come from the shoe store with a new pair of white bucs.

"That shot sho' did break 'at o' bull from suckin' eggs, didn't it?" allowed one viewer.

"Yep, that vetnerry sho' cured him, meanness and all!" echoed another.

I don't actually think that the wildness was surgically removed along with the corns. But that bull sure did calm down a lot after the episode, according to Mr. Boudreaux and all the neighbors. All the neighbors except Mutt. I found out later that he wasn't a cowboy at all, but just an apprentice cutter at a potato chip factory. He just liked to dress up like a cowboy on his day off. We sure broke him from sucking eggs!

15

Four kinds of pickup truck owners

AFTER many months of waiting, wishing and watching for the best possible deal, I finally have done it. I have obtained a new pickup truck! It's not the red and white, four-wheel-drive job that I really wanted, but I am right satisfied with the one that I have settled for.

While I was trying to decide exactly what kind of truck that I could afford, I also made a study of the types and appearances of pickup trucks and the types of people who drive them.

My research indicates that the pickup truck industry is enjoying unprecedented popularity and that the growth of truck ownership is mushrooming, similar to cheese sales. In addition, I have observed that there are about four distinct groups of people who own and drive them.

Farmers: Obviously, trucks and farmers were made for each other, kind of like moon pies were made for RC colas, or vice versa.

Farmers probably were the first owners of pickups and always should get first priority in times of truck shortages. In fact, it might be a good idea to require nonfarmers to present a signed permission slip from the ASCS office or the county agent in order to buy a truck in locales where there aren't enough to go around.

A farmer's truck usually is dirty, dusty and will have a considerable amount of grease smeared at various spots over its external surface. The grill always is messed up, the hood flops up and down while driving down a rough road, and there are mighty few hubcaps on the wheels of the farmers' trucks that I have seen.

The bed usually contains junk items of great variety. Drink cans, milk cartons, leftover sorghum seed, much hay twine, several empty sacks and used plastic O.B.

sleeves always are there. You may see plowpoints, empty chewing tobacco sacks, a worn-out tire and a dead calf. The tailgate always has a big round dent in the top where a pine tree has been butted firmly while the daydreaming driver was backing the vehicle with the gate down.

Practically, it is impossible for a visitor to be able to sit comfortably in the passenger seat, even if he can get in the door. The seat and floorboard will contain fencing items, nails, syringes and needles, and wooden stakes or iron pipes. There usually are old DHIA records strowed about, four or five flashlights and numerous bangle tags and neck chains rattling about on the floor.

When cranked, the thing can be heard by at least three farmer neighbors down the road. The horn won't blow, nor will the radio play consistently. Even though there only are 30,000 miles on the speedometer, it is hard to believe that the truck ever was new.

In spite of all the dirt, dents, junk and noise, these trucks seem to be able to run forever. If called upon, they would carry that farmer dependably from coast to coast or from pole to pole.

Pseudofarmers: This category includes all those individuals who always have wanted to farm but never have had nerve to try. Many veterinarians belong in this group, as do other people from all walks of life. Many factory workers, chimney sweeps, pole climbers and encyclopedia salesmen like to drive their pickups down to the co-op after work and buy a sack of dog food, just so they can throw it in the back and drive off.

Trucks owned by pseudofarmers usually are fairly clean, since they have more time to run them through the automatic car wash than do real farmers. Also, there aren't a whole lot of dents and caved-in fenders.

Many pseudofarmers buy one of those $10,000 trucks for no other reason than to play farmer and to haul two or three loads of firewood a year in the thing. 'Course a lot of these people cut the wrong kind of wood since they don't know the difference between a sweetgum and red oak tree. I saw a guy just the other day, and he was so proud of the load of half rotten pine he had on his 1983 short bed Nissan.

Other uses include hauling little leaguers, taking sofas and chairs to the upholsterer, hauling off the garbage and taking broken bicycles to the bike shop. Some carry a burlap sack of unknown material and a bale of hay in the bed, in order to look more realistic.

Hunters: The road by my house is wrapped up with trucks during deer hunting season. Starting about 5 a.m. on opening day, the line of truck headlights looks like a never ending funeral procession. Most of these trucks are four-wheel drive types with huge cleaty tires that have big white letters on the side.

In order to qualify for this category, there must be a gun rack over the rear window, and it must be chock full of expensive and scoped deer rifles. A minimum of two tobacco chawed and unshaven quasi-hunters should be seated inside the cab.

The big difference between a hunter's truck and a farmer's truck is that the former usually is beautifully covered with mud, but has no dents. Also, there is more evidence of alcohol consumption, in general, in the bed of hunters' trucks. There frequently will be empty beer cans, hamburger wrappers and fried chicken boxes in there, also. In addition, when you meet them on the road, deer hunters won't wave at you like farmers do. A real farmer waves at everybody he meets while driving because it might be the banker that he is meeting. Friendliness goes a long way when you go into the community bank, with hat in hand, to "make arrangements" with a scowling loan officer.

Mystery owners: This is the fourth and last category of pickup truck drivers. These are the people who drive trucks for no apparent reason, other than the influence of TV. I think they must have seen the ad where the truck climbs a mountain of rocks and they think that owning a truck makes them more macho.

These people put those plastic liner beds in the back and never, never haul anything in the bed except a sack of groceries. They continually are taking a clean diaper out of the glove compartment and wiping fingerprints and particles of dust off the paint job. They always wear gloves when driving, and make a big to-do about starting the vehicle. Some act as if they are 747 pilots and go through a long checklist before taking off.

There is one of these "mystery owners" who lives down the road from me. I think he is a math or physics professor, or some other brilliant basic scientist, because he has a funny looking goatee and dresses like some of the professors I had years ago in my pre-vet science courses. He wears an old gray tweed coat, khaki pants and sneakers, regardless of the situation. He is really particular about his no-chrome and no-frills imported truck.

A few weeks ago when I ran out of gas down the road, he came along and offered me a ride. Just as I opened the door and prepared to sit, he stopped me.

"Hey, wait!" he said with a start. "Don't sit! You have soiled trousers. What's that dried green material on your thigh?"

"I guess it's cow manure, since I was just at the dairy," I answered nonchalantly, as I quickly brushed at a faint spot.

"Oh my goodness!" he screamed. "There's some on your boots, also! Let me put something over the seat and floorboard so they won't get soiled."

As he meticulously arranged several layers of the Wall Street Journal over the interior of the truck, I stood there sheepishly wishing that he had not stopped and offered me a ride. I really wasn't that dirty!

Nevertheless, I sat carefully as he took me by the service station. When I got out, he removed the newspapers, threw them in the trash and started brushing the seats off with a whisk broom. I'm sure he fumigated it later.

Trucks owned by these mysterious types **always** are spotless, shiny and retain that new smell for years. These owners don't "sell" those trucks after a few years. Instead, they let someone adopt them as if the trucks were Cabbage Patch dolls.

Several years ago, I was lucky enough to adopt one of these trucks, but not before the guy interviewed me and checked me out very carefully. He made me agree to carry out all sorts of maintenance procedures before I drove off.

Pickup trucks are kind of like pocket knives, except that trucks cost a whole lot more. They both are necessary items, both are sources of pride to their owners, and owners of both continually are arguing about which brand or make is the best. All persons, regardless of age or gender, need a couple of toys. I reckon trucks and knives fill the bill!

16

"You just can't get there from here"

VETERINARIANS know where all the farms are! They also are pretty well up to date on who owns what farm or who rents what and where various citizens reside.

After vets have been in practice in a particular locale for several years, they could be a great source of information for the census takers, the UPS man or fledgling politicians who are searching out key citizens in a particular township. I figure it takes a minimum of about three years of busy farm call practice to learn the area.

When I first opened up my practice, the only person I knew in the county was my friend, the county agent. He had encouraged me to come there, had answered many agricultural questions and had kind of run interference for me.

As the calls started coming in, I didn't realize how difficult it was going to be just finding where that sick cow was located. In that county, it appeared that roads had not been planned. They had just been cut through anywhere that looked like a good place. So the result was a maze of curvy, crisscrossing passageways, most of which had no name or number. Few were paved, or "blacktopped," as we often call the paved farm-to-market roads.

"Could you tell me where your place is?" I would ask a farmer when he or she would call in about a sick cow.

"Well, we're just a half a mile past the old Smith place," they'd say.

"Well, I'm kind of new here and I'm not real familiar with the area yet," I'd apologize. "Could you tell me which direction you are from here?"

Once we'd established whether the farm was north, south, east or west from my office, then I'd try to plot it out on a big county map that I had.

Another problem that still occurs is that someone will call in and ask for vet service. When the office person asks for directions, the caller will not want to give them.

"Doc's been here before. He knows the way!" the caller will say.

That may be true, but if the farm is outside the practice area, or if that particular farmer has several farms, then problems can occur.

Nighttime calls are the worst for directions.

"Come to the third dirt road to the left past the old Toxey schoolhouse. Come to the big oak tree across from the campground. Turn right. Come about four miles. You'll see a green car parked in front of a brown trailer. The horse is behind the trailer."

Hidden by kudzu . . .

What they failed to say was that the old schoolhouse was torn down in 1965, and the dirt road is hidden by kudzu vines. There is a white oak, a red oak and a water oak across from the campground, and there are three dirt roads there. Then, how can you tell the color of a car and a trailer in pitch black dark? There are several cars and several trailers on that road.

One night I became hopelessly lost while trying to find a colicky horse in the neighboring state. I always have been against stopping and asking for directions, but this time I just had to do it. I knew that I was right on the state line since the place where I stopped was a honky-tonk called "The First Chance." It was one of those places where they issue you a knife or brass knuckles, if you don't have a weapon, when you walk in the door.

The roughnecks and rednecks around the bar numbered about a dozen, and their appearance was enough to chill the spine of the toughest hockey player. In fact, the Los Angeles Raiders probably would have eased up to the bar with fear and trepidation.

"Can any of y'all tell me where Junior Smith's place is around here?" I asked boldly.

"Who wants to know?" asked a bearded outlaw roughly as he turned and pointed his cantilevered belly in my general direction. Another guy finished his beer and crushed the metal can into a watch-fob-sized mass with one hand.

He grinned a toothless grin.

The whole crowd then turned to stare at the uninvited stranger.

"I'm the vet, and one of Junior's horses is bad sick. He asked me to come over and see about it. I just can't seem to find his place," I said. I figured that telling them that I was a doctor would keep them from wanting to challenge me to a fight.

You kill Fred's cow?

"You the same vet that killed Fred's cow?" bristled a runt-sized guy at the end of the bar.

"Naw, sir, it wasn't me, must've been Dr. McDaniel over at Red Hill," I said, pleadingly. Maybe I had made a mistake by owning up to being a vet.

One of the more sober of the group was trying to be helpful, so he came over and tried to explain how to get to Junior's place.

"Go down the blacktop towards the creek. Just past the creek is a gravel road to the left. Go down that road till you come to a crossroad, then . . ."

"Naw, that ain't right, Buck," slurred another drinker. "It'd be better if he'd go back the other way and come in by the rock quarry."

"Both of you are wrong," growled the bartender. "That bridge is out over the Moss Plantation, so he'd better come in by the loggin' road through Rudder Hill Hunting Club land."

"Look," said a fourth guy, "you just can't get there from here. He'll have to go back to Butler and start from there."

"Thanks," I allowed, and I fled out the door. As I made my way over beer cans and broken bottles, I could hear them arguing loudly over how to get to Junior's place. Bar stools were beginning to crash, and then I heard a bottle hit the side of the building.

When I pulled onto the road, two scuffling bodies came hurtling out of the barroom door, amid flailing arms and flying cowboy hats. All I had asked for were simple directions to a farm, but innocently I had instigated a minor war! Since that time, I have avoided taverns even though desperately needing directions.

My wife is by far the best "direction getter" that I have

seen. The other day I found an old note she made. It was about how to get to a particular farm.

"Go 12.6 miles south of Doggett Hardware Store. On the left side of the road there will be a yellow sign that says, 'Honey for Sale!' Turn left on that dirt road. Come down that road exactly six miles. On the right side of the road you will see a white aluminum-sided house with a red roof. Just past the house will be a two-acre pasture with a 12-year-old racking horse in it. Turn right just beyond the pasture on a creek gravel road. Come up that road until you see a shuck basket turned upside down on the right side of the road. Stop there. Look to your right. There will be a hog lot about 50 paces down the hill. There will be three white hogs and one red hog in a pen. The red hog's name is Sam. He is sick. Leave a note under the shuck basket — Jan.

"P.S.: Don't drive too fast. Be careful. I love you! — J."

Now that is what I call good directions!

17

There are advantages to getting older

IT'S STRANGE and frustrating how older farmers sometimes won't believe what a young veterinarian says. When
I was fresh out of veterinary school, that was hard to
understand and accept.

"Sir, I'm afraid this nice steer has got the blackleg," I'd
tell a crusty, frowning and always-doubting 90-year-old
cattleman.

"Aw, boy," he'd growl. "This here ain't blackleg!
They're **dead** when they git the blackleg! This calf's just
got a swoll'up leg cause that fool mule kicked him. Where's
my gun, I'm gonna clear out aroun' here, startin' with that
devilish plug mule!"

"I don't know, Sir," I'd tremble, "there sure is a lot of
crepitation and swelling under this skin here, and it smells
like rancid butter just like the book says. The temperature
is 105°, and you neglected to vaccinate just like the book
says."

"The book, my achin' back!" he'd explode. "You young
wet-behind-the-ears chaps don't know nothin' but what's in
a book! Wait'll you've been around as long as I have, and
you'll know somethin' about stock."

"Yessir."

Another time I had a phone call from a very proper elderly lady.

"Is the Doctuh in?" her proper voice questioned when I
answered the telephone.

"Yes'm," I replied. "I'm the Doctor. May I help you?"

"Oh, you sound so young. I thought you were one of his
young children," she said.

I cringed and gripped the phone tighter.

"Perhaps you can help me anyway," she continued. "I
am Miss Sue Beesley at the old Beesley farm. We've had

the misfortune to have one of our fine cows show up this morning with a swollen foot. I'm certain that she has foot and mouth disease."

My ears perked up when she came out with that foreign disease. "Well, Ma'am," I said in my most diplomatic manner, "that disease is mighty rare in the U.S., and I expect that you might be dealing with something a lot more common, like foot rot or a foot injury."

"Young man," she replied curtly, "I am a registered nurse and am well informed about medical matters. The symptoms that I have observed in my cow are consistent with the dreaded scourge, foot and mouth disease!"

"Yes'm." I never argue with people who are certain they know more about my job than I do. Besides, I don't like arguing. If Miss Beesley wanted her cow to have foot and mouth disease, it was okay with me. I wondered if she realized that I would have to report it immediately to the head honcho at the state department of agriculture.

"Young man," she said as she continued her lecture, "you obviously are very inexperienced. I have lived a long time, have a Merck Manual, a USDA Yearbook on cattle diseases and my son-in-law is a chiropractor. I am no dummy! I'm not calling you to pass the time of day. I will expect you on my premises within one hour, or I will hold you personally responsible for any cattle of mine that expire."

"Yes'm." We don't talk back to our elders in the South, regardless of how badly we want to.

Upon arrival at the farm, I was treated to more lecturing on the pathogenesis of foot and mouth disease and the rampant effect it surely would have upon her stock. She failed to mention, however, that the ailment hadn't been diagnosed in the country for years.

As I moved to catch the wild, three-legged lame cow with a rope, Miss Beesley shifted gears swiftly and went into a long-winded episode on proper restraint and how young people didn't have a way with cows like the older folks did.

When I tried to pick up the sore foot and immediately got stomped, she lectured me on the proper way to do that, too. More of the same followed when I checked out the hoof wall and coronary band. She was back on foot and mouth disease now and was on a roll.

I was learning so much pathology from her that I almost

was sorry when I found the roofing nail in the cow's foot.

"Ma'am," I said in between cow kicks and when she paused to get her breath, "we don't have foot and mouth disease here; we've got nail-in-the-foot disease. See here!"

Suddenly she was quiet. It was as if she had been struck dumb. A few head nods and mumbles were all that I got from her for the remainder of the visit.

After she had written me a check and was tearing it out of her checkbook, she stared at me.

"Well, I guess you must be a right smart older than you look and sound like over the phone," she said in a disappointed tone.

Now that I have some gray hair, knobby fingers, a hunched-over back and have sacrificed most of my productive years working at dusty, man-killing sale barns, people tend to listen to me more than they did 25 or 30 years ago.

Just the other day, Bud and I were riding in his old, worn-out pickup truck through his heifer pasture. We saw this one heifer lagging behind the rest of the group. She had swollen rear legs, enlarged joints, a jugular pulse and a dry nose.

"Heifer's got endocarditis, Bud," I said matter-of-factly. "She's got a growth on one of her heart valves big as a biscuit. Must've had an infected navel a while back."

Did he doubt my word? Did he look askance and purse his lips? Did he question my windshield diagnostic methods? No sirree!

"Doc, I'll bet you are right," he agreed. "She did have a swollen navel when she was small."

Now, it's the young folks who think I am too old to practice veterinary medicine properly. When I took my vet students back to Bud's the next day to treat the heifer, they were aghast at my inside-the-truck diagnosis.

They snickered, actually laughed aloud, and told me that I was wrong and old-fashioned.

"What's her CBC look like?" demanded one.

"Have you run an EKG?" sneered another.

"Is the fibrinogen elevated?"

"Have you ausculted her cardiovascular system?"

They all shook their heads in disbelief as I got my lariat from under the seat.

"Just clam it up, you young, wet-behind-the-ears children. Sooner or later you, too, will learn to use your eyes, ears, hands and brain at the same time," I preached. "You can't be running EKG's and all those fancy tests on every cow you see!"

"Sir, you just can't look out a car window and make a diagnosis," said the most diplomatic of the group. "You've just got to do a series of lab tests before you can tell. You are kind of behind the times."

I can't understand it! Just yesterday I was too young to know anything, and today I'm too old! Where was I when I was middle-aged and knew it all?

18

The day the chute turned over

I WOULD like to shake hands with the gentleman who designed or invented the first portable livestock holding squeeze chute.

By making it possible to restrain wild cattle safely for routine veterinary work, such as dehorning, vaccination and pregnancy checking, the device has made my life much easier. Without the chute, there would be a lot more roping and hemming beasts up between the hammer mill and corn crib for various veterinary matters.

There have been times, though, when I thought that squeeze chutes were going to be responsible for my premature checking in at the great veterinary clinic in the sky.

I had been in my own practice for about six months when I decided that I just had to have a chute. A handyman in a nearby town built an occasional one in his spare time, so I talked him into building one for me.

His design was simple. The chute was quite lengthy, long enough to accommodate two adult cows, one behind the other. Since the sides were made of 2-inch by 12-inch pine lumber, the cows couldn't see out the sides when it was backed up to a cracked open barn door. All the cows could see was an opening in the front, and sometimes one would go into the chute out of curiosity, or perhaps thinking she was going to escape. Then another cow would follow the first one in, not knowing what was in store for her.

The front headgate, or neck squeeze as we often called it, also was made of 2-inch by 12-inch lumber. Stationary at the bottom, it opened up at the top in the shape of a "V." To close the headgate, the operator just pulled down on a rope, which was attached to a vertical metal bar, some cables and turnbuckles, and this action closed the two boards, trapping the animal's head. Care had to be taken though, when pulling on the rope, to be sure that the operator's head was not in the line of descent of the metal bar.

When it finally arrived, I was so proud of my new "toy." In order to show off how easily it made working cattle, I lined up the meanest, wildest herd of Brahman-blooded cattle in the county to test for Bang's disease, dehorn and deworm. I was going to show those people how cattle should be handled.

On the appointed morning, I drove back and forth through town three times with the chute trailing behind my truck, just showing off. I waved, tooted the horn and grinned at the local hardware store sitters, as they scratched their heads and peered at each other, wondering what kind of combat equipment Doc was dragging behind his white Chevrolet. Had I known the surprises that were in store for me while working and pulling that chute, my confident grin would have turned quickly to a slack jawed frown.

Arriving at the Brahman wild cow ranch, I quickly and expertly backed the two-wheeled chute up to the barn door. Backing the chute is difficult for some, but, quite frankly, it is child's play after backing a four-wheel manure spreader into the hallway of a narrow Tennessee mule barn.

Pleasantries were exchanged, compliments offered on the new purchase and boot laces tightened. Then I announced that I was ready to catch a cow.

Presently, I saw a wild cow streaking for the head gate and a devilish smirk of a smile elevated my upper lip. Just as she hit the headgate, I yanked down with all my might on the rope. I vaguely remember a noise that sounded like a sonic boom, and, way off somewhere, I heard some teeth click together. In my exuberance, I had forgotten about the steel bar above my head. When it came down, it put a furrow in my scalp deep enough for planting cotton.

I was told later that it took two buckets of pond water to revive me. The next thing that I recollect was the feeling of sutures being squeaked through the scalp laceration and trying to explain what a squeeze chute was to the emergency room attendants.

The chute stayed on the mean and wild Brahman cow ranch for several days after the auspicious initiation.

Another close call occurred on a hot July afternoon while

returning from testing cows in the neighboring county to the north. As usual, I was late and I had the truck and chute barreling down the road a couple dozen miles or so over the speed limit. Suddenly, I hit a pothole in the narrow farm-to-market road and the truck surged forward. Knowing that something was wrong, I glanced into the rearview mirror, just in time to see the chute upside down and coming at the truck. I jammed the accelerator to the floor and barely shot out of range, just in time to see it flip over into the ditch and plow up about 40 feet of a healthy stand of kudzu.

As I reversed the truck and neared the scene of destruction, a motorist slowed down and stopped. The chute, laying sideways, had great gobs of fertile mud dripping from all available points, splintered boards pointing crazily at all angles and both wheels were still whirling crookedly.

"What happened?" asked the wide-eyed motorist, ignorantly.

"Aw, I think it's either out of gas or it's just got a dead batt'ry," I joked.

The motorist didn't appreciate my attempt at humor as he sped away, throwing gravel and chopped-up kudzu vines all over the scene with his recapped tires.

The chute spent a week in the intensive care section of the chute hospital and was almost as good as new after that, except that the headgate never did close quite as smoothly. The accident did modify my hookup system from a self-locking Farmall pin to a ball-type hitch, and I haven't lost another chute since.

One of my most amusing chute incidents occurred one Sunday afternoon. Sunday is family day at our place. But this one time, a weekend farmer and bootlegger talked me into bringing my chute to his place to work some cows. I hastily set up the chute but forgot to chain it to the corral. The first patient to volunteer was the bull. He was a 7-year-old Polled Hereford that weighed about a ton, but he entered the squeeze with the speed and enthusiasm of a hopped up weanling.

Bull and chute gained speed . . .

He hit the headgate and it closed cleanly on his massive neck. However, he was so strong that he started pushing

71

and gaining footing on the ground since the chute had no floor. As he pushed, the chute began to move, slowly at first. But, as he eased down the hill, both bull and chute gained speed and presently a weird and amusing, yet serious, condition existed. The bull would run with the chute gripped tightly against his neck. He then would stop to rest briefly and allow us to catch up to him before charging off again. In the meantime, both the farmer and I were running about waving our hands and shouting insults to the bull.

"Stop, you old fool!" or "Be still, you old heathen, and I'll turn you loose!"

He would retaliate by slinging his head and bellowing loudly. Amidst all the yelling and bellowing, the patient finally jammed the chute up against a pine stump and his joy ride was over.

The bull was released from his predicament but mine was continuing. The chute appeared to be sinking in a marsh. We quickly obtained all the log chains we could find in the neighborhood and pulled the thing out with a G John Deere. When it came to rest on high ground, I hooked it up and prepared to leave.

"The Master finds ways of punishing folks for trying to dehorn cows on Sunday," I preached as I got into the truck.

"Doc, wait! Doc, don't leave. We'll get 'em back up. It won't take but another hour . . ." the stunned sinner's voice trailed off as I drove away.

19

Carney Sam

CARNEY Sam Jenkins won't be sitting on his favorite nail keg at the country store this morning.

Carney Sam, a great southern American, a natural homespun philosopher and a good honest man, passed away last night. At this very moment he is swapping yarns, probably even telling tales with St. Peter or St. Paul or whoever is the official tall tale teller at that great country store just outside the pearly gates.

I first became acquainted with Carney Sam late one rainy autumn afternoon while returning home from a sick cow call. Most roads back then weren't paved and the one I was traveling that day was mostly holes and mud, with an occasional sprinkling of gravel. Through the drizzle and fog I saw him walking slowly, a red plaid flannel shirt, a Funk's G Hybrid cap and engineer's boots. He was always attired in this particular garb, regardless of the season.

"Goin' to town?" I yelled, splashing up beside him.

He eyed me suspiciously, glanced at the mud-covered white truck with the long whipping two-way radio antenna and drawled, "Ah reckon so, ain't gettin' nowhere lack this."

Trying to make conversation during the ride to town was difficult, since it was obvious to him that I was a new resident in the area and thus was not yet to be trusted. Any outsiders coming into Choctaw County first must be exposed to and successfully negotiate the scrutiny of certain native residents before being granted probationary acceptance.

"Fool with cows do ye?" he queried, as he sniffed at the aroma of fresh, lush fescue cow manure that permeated the interior of the truck.

"Yessir, I'm the new veterinarian in the county," I replied with a certain degree of pride and self-confidence.

"Ah'm sort of a veterinary myself," he declared, matter-of-factly. "Ah'm the one they come an'git when their stock is sick."

Well, there it was. He actually admitted to being the community's home-made veterinarian. Previous to my arrival, there never had been a genuine, registered D.V.M. in the area, so they had to make do with what they had. Some of these men did a good job; some didn't.

Stunned look . . .

"So you are the man I've heard about," I exclaimed. He could see the stunned look on my face when I realized that he would likely be my chief competitor. I wanted to lecture him on state board examinations, licensing fees, malpractice insurance and all the other things required of veterinary practitioners, but even then I knew enough not to get into an argument with him.

"Yep, I like foolin' with them beasts. I try to he'p my neighbors with their stock any way I kin."

At that very moment I made up my mind that Carney Sam and I were not only going to get along with each other, but we were also going to become friends and perhaps even have some degree of respect for each other.

The remainder of the trip to town was uneventful, except that I kept noticing him scrunching down into his seat occasionally, and closing his eyes tightly as if in prayer. When I let him out in front of the Piggly Wiggly, he said, "Boy, listen heah! You treat folks right around heah, and you'll do arright. Treat 'em wrong, an' they'll hurt you." As an afterthought he blurted out, "You drive too fast!"

Carney Sam's hangout, or executive office as we called it, was at Mrs. Ruby McCord's store. The nail keg just to the right of the hoop cheese was his personal domain. Somehow, when he sat upon that keg, he became an expert on the world's problems. In addition to conducting earth shaking seminars from there, he also could whittle, spit into the wood box, feed cheese to the cats around the stove and get the first view of all intruders that drove up and came into the store.

He had a basic philosophy about life that contradicted his own lifestyle. He said that 10 acres of a rocky hillside cotton field, 25 acres of bottomland corn so thick with

74

buckgrass that you couldn't tell where the rows were, and a quarter mile of fencerow overgrown with thorn trees would cure everything from juvenile delinquency to asthma.

As the months and years went by, our friendship prospered, in spite of our differences. Often, I would go by Mrs. McCord's store on the pretense of getting a pint of milk to ease my ulcer, just to get Carney Sam to ride with me and help me out with herd work.

About the time Russia's Premier Kruschev was banging his shoe on a table in the U.N., we were testing a herd of cows for brucellosis. As I clamped a silver tag in a bellowing cow's ear, Carney exclaimed, "Ole Kruschev oughta have one o' them thangs in his ear!" As I took a jugular blood sample with a 15-gauge needle, he vowed, "If they'd let me git aholt o' them Russians with a few of them needles, I'd cure all this here war mess, too!" He always pronounced the word Russians with a long "u."

His expertise in foreign affairs was not limited to the Soviet Union. He could and would tell you what was wrong with our European allies or could analyze the critical situation in the Middle East as quickly as the most learned university professor.

Naturally, local politics were just child's play to him. He could tell you months in advance who would be running for sheriff, the school board, tax assessor or district attorney. Shoot, he could even tell you who was even thinking about being a candidate. After election day, he would tell you how everybody had voted and why, plus what had been paid to whom to get their support. He would have made the analysis of the national television networks look silly in comparison.

He was a master of predicting how severe winter would be, how hot the summer would be, or how many deer would be killed on opening day at Rudder Hill Hunting Club.

Still, in spite of all his knowledge and expertise, he couldn't understand some of the most basic concepts of animal husbandry. One day I stopped by the store to swap lies with him. He was whittling and spitting.

"Where you been, Doc?" he asked.

"Aw, I've been up at Mr. Lanier's place pregnancy checking cows," I replied.

"What's the matter; ain't he got no bull?" he asked in amazement, with a strange look on his face.

After a couple of unsuccessful attempts at explaining to him the reasons for fertility exams and getting rid of unproductive cow boarders, I gave up. Convincing him of the need for a controlled breeding season, utilizing A.I., and having a small calving pasture would be nigh impossible. In fact, it would have been easier to convince a locust post imbedded in four feet of limestone rock.

People like Carney Sam don't come along every day. The advantage of dealing with less complex individuals is that you always know where you stand with them. When they don't like something, they say so. There is no double talk or wordy mumbo jumbo. Their word is their bond and people like Carney Sam Jenkins stick to their word until the cows come home. We have too few of them anymore, and I miss them very much.

20

"You've fixed Spot?"

I COULD see the cows penned behind Mr. Mabry's barn waiting for me as the truck sloshed through the cold February mud of the driveway. At least half the cows were wearing "yokes." A "yoke" is a long, vertical, narrow Y-shaped device worn on the necks of certain cantankerous bovines. Purpose of the yoke is to prevent the animal from escaping through the fence when she is seeking the grazing which always is greener on the other side.

There are store-bought yokes and homemade yokes. Nearly all of the dozens that I have observed are of the homemade variety. To create one, the cow owner tromps out into the woods, with axe in hand, and seeks out a tree or sapling which has a branch with the proper shape. The best one resembles a tuning fork. It should be four or five feet long, depending upon the size of the cow, after it has been chopped out of the sapling. The bark should be skinned off the thing and any knotty spots smoothed off with your sharp and always clean pocket knife.

The cow's neck is fitted into the "V" part of the yoke with the open part at the top. Then, some wire or plowline is stretched across the top of the neck and tied to the two vertically ascending yoke parts. The wire or rope should be liberally wrapped with a burlap sack or rags swiped from under the sink. If it works correctly, the long device catches the top and bottom strand of the barbed wire when the hungry cow tries to push through the fence.

When I saw Mr. Mabry working on the well pump and when I noticed the flat rear tire on the Allis-Chalmers, I should have realized that he was in no mood for frivolity. But I didn't think.

"The snakes bad out here?" I asked cheerfully, as he approached where I was standing.

"No, I don't reckon," he replied. "Why?"

"Well, I just noticed that most of those cows are carrying sticks," I said, looking in the direction of the 30 or so bovines.

He didn't respond to my attempt at humor. I noticed that his face was changing slowly from an off-white color to the shade of a just-pulled spring radish. After about an eight-second delay, I smiled very weakly and offered an explanation.

"I'm sorry," I declared, "I was just joking. I didn't mean anything by it."

"Well, let me tell you something, four eyes," he exploded. "If you're coming out here to be a smart aleck, you can just get back in your old truck and get off my property."

"Aw I'm sorry, I just . . ."

"Yeah, just go! Git! I can get another vet to worm my cows." Then he stomped off in a huff. He was so mad I could almost hear him sizzling as he kicked mud and frozen clods with his five-buckle overshoes.

I was afraid that he was going to get his shotgun, so I did as he suggested. As I turned around and headed back out the driveway, I could see him tinkering with the water pipes and glaring at me in disgust.

"Why? Why did I do it?" I asked myself as I sheepishly retreated back down the road. I had violated one of the cardinal rules of veterinary practice — Be courteous to everyone! I swore that I would try to do better.

A few hours later a lady came into the clinic with her dog. She was dressed in the latest fashions and even had three or four red fox hides draped around her shoulders and working down one arm. The dog was a small brownish type with lots of fur. It was obvious that the lady spent a lot of time combing and brushing her pet.

When she placed the patient upon the examination table, I blundered again.

"Nice little feist dog you have here," I declared, as I patted the dog's head and checked its gums.

"Feist?" she screamed. "This is no feist! I'll have you know that this is a full-blooded, registered, champion Pomeranian! What kind of vet are you? You don't even know a Pom from a cur!"

With that she snatched the perfume-saturated canine

from the table and exited the exam room with great acceleration, her fox skins streaming behind her like a hairy scarf. Seconds later, she scratched off in her Cadillac and headed toward the country club.

I said the wrong thing again! When would I ever learn? I immediately reviewed the breeds of dogs and memorized their approximate weights, distinguishing characteristics and the type of persons that would likely own them.

"Whitney, bring up that little black and white squirrel dog to be spayed," I yelled into the back, still thinking about the two mistakes in judgment I had made that day. I couldn't waste any time worrying about dumb things I had done though, I had too many other things to do.

While operating on the dog, an elderly couple drove up, slowly got out of their old pickup truck and came into the waiting room.

"We've come to get Spot, our little black and white squirrel dog. We left her here for boarding," I heard them tell Mrs. Lee, our receptionist.

Spayed wrong dog . . .

A wave of panic raced through my brain, and a cold chill bolted up my spine as I halted my needle and catgut in mid-air. Could it be that I was spaying the wrong dog? Don't mistakes and accidents come in threes?

Minutes later, when Whitney presented the couple with a black and white dog, I heard the bad news.

" That's not Spot, but she does look a whole lot like her. Spot has a short tail," the lady said.

I raised the drape slowly and peeked underneath. Just as I thought, there was the short tail. I had operated on the wrong dog! The third mistake in one day!

There was nothing to do but go out and admit my mistake and face the music. I took a deep breath and strode to the door, still wearing my surgical garb.

"Mr. and Mrs. Thomas," I began, "we have two almost identical dogs in the clinic. One is in for boarding, and the other one is in to be spayed."

"Yessir, I see," the lady said, puzzled. "But what does that have to do with Spot?"

"I have spayed Spot," I blurted.

"What! You've fixed Spot so she can't ever have puppies?'' exclaimed Mrs. Thomas, with hands over mouth.

"Yes, Ma'am, that's correct," I replied, "but she's doing just fine."

For a brief period, there was complete silence, except for the barking of the dogs back in the kennel and the soft trickle of sweat running down my back. I didn't know whether Spot's folks were going to sue or have me arrested or what. I do know that as they stood there open-mouthed, I considered running away to Egypt. Finally, Mr. Thomas spoke.

"Well, Doctor, we've been considering getting her fixed anyway," he said smiling. "I'm glad you went ahead and did it."

"That's right," Mrs. Thomas allowed. "Now we won't always have to be penning her up and worrying about her having a batch of unwanted puppies."

"When can we pick her up?" he asked.

I just stood there, stunned and shaken, trying to get my tongue to work.

"Doctor, when can we pick her up?"

"Oh, yes," I finally said, "tomorrow or the next day will be fine."

I went back into the surgery and nervously finished suturing the skin incision. From the surgery window, I could see Mr. and Mrs. Thomas smiling broadly as they got into their vehicle and left.

What a day! After the events of the day, I wondered if I was in the right line of work. Perhaps I was not suited for dealing with people and would be better off working with timber, painting bridges or working on a shrimp boat. I decided to get out of the clinic for a while and do some thinking. Maybe I'd run by the house and see how Jan and the kids were doing.

"Y'all having fun?" I said, as I walked into the house.

"Having fun? HA!" Jan exclaimed. "Tommy came home from nursery school running a high fever, and Lisa has cried all day with her ears. The washing machine broke down a while ago, and now I've just burned supper! And now you come in here asking if I'm having fun! Sometimes I wish you and I could swap jobs for just one day. Then you'd see what I have to go through!"

In seconds I was in the truck, heading back to the clinic.

I would just have to learn how to do a better job of talking with animal owners. Housework and raising children were much too difficult.

Since that difficult day in 1961, I have studied client relations and how to communicate better with the people for whom I work. I believe that I have improved slightly since then.

21

A classic case of rock music overload

IN MY opinion, one of life's greatest pleasures is the enjoyment of good country music. It is soothing, has a nice beat to it, and it will tell you a story. The tale may be genuinely sad, sometimes sarcastically amusing and often hilariously funny.

I've always thought this type of music was created by The Master primarily for busy veterinarians who spend a large portion of their time driving from farm to farm in pickup trucks or muddy two-door sedans. Between calls the stresses of dealing with those farm crises can be significantly reduced by listening to songs like, "My Wife's Gonna Hire a Wino To Redecorate Our Home" or "It's Hard To Be Humble."

My favorite time of day to enjoy country music is early in the morning while driving sleepily to an emergency or herd work. The cool, early morning air is so fresh and healthful, and the small towns are so peaceful and quiet.

All the time the strains of Jerry Reed and Porter Waggoner and Willie Nelson are wailing about how somebody done 'em wrong or how much they miss the woman who left 'em on account of their drinking and carousing. By the time I get to the farm I'm in a real good, mellow mood because I realize how fortunate I am to not have all those knotty and trying problems. If the calves aren't up or the downer cow is over on the back 40, it doesn't seem quite as bad as it might be.

Most of the dairies that we visit have their parlor radios turned to the local country station. Most allow as how the cows are more contented and thus give more milk when exposed to "Highway 40 Blues" and "Cadillac Johnson."

Back in the winter one night, a dairyman called. He was in a frenzy as he breathed heavily into the phone.

"Doc, can you come out here?" he heaved. "My cows were off a thousand pounds today and have been off a good bit the last few days."

"Reckon it can wait till daylight?" I asked sleepily. After all, I was asleep in my easy chair, absorbing the news by osmosis.

"Tell you what," I said. "Let me dash out first thing in the morning and we'll take a look."

"Awright, Doc, but please come as soon as you can," he pleaded. "Don't stop by the donut shop or you won't get here 'til way up in the day!"

After I finally got to sleep, I dreamed of all kinds of problems the dairyman might have. In my dream I could envision all sorts of weird and devastating health problems descending upon his previously healthy herd. Foot and mouth disease was rampant, PCB's, aflatoxins and arsenic were contaminating the grain mix and stray voltage was coursing through the spotless parlor in erratic but powerful surges. The milkers were calmly and uncaringly jerking teat cups off stomping and wildly kicking cows whose teats and udders were a mass of ugly blisters and sores.

Meanwhile, the dairyman was standing on the front steps of the parlor, with eyes rolled towards the heavens as he ripped and pulled at the few hairs he had left on top of his anemic skull. Immediately behind him was his aproned wife who struck a disgusted pose with hands on hips and with smoke boiling out of both ears.

I was awakened from my nightmarish sleep by the clock radio as Charlie Pride lustily rendered a country tear-jerker about how life would be if a specific young lady accepted his proposal.

As I made my way through town, lights were open at the donut shop, and the truck strained and tugged mightily to turn in at the curb for a fresh dozen or so. With much willpower, though, I overcame the strenuous efforts of the vehicle and quickly made my way on to the farm.

Driving up beside the parlor, I knew something was amiss. A new man with a walking stick was in the holding pen trying to make reluctant cows go into the parlor.

"Reckon why those cows don't want to be milked?" I pondered, as the guy cracked a Holstein in the forehead.

About that time I heard an awful sound. There was screaming and hollering in weird unknown tongues coming from inside the parlor. My first thought was that someone either had been severely bitten by a vicious cow or perhaps had thoughtlessly sat down on the red hot heater.

Rushing into the parlor, I discovered two bored milkers and one vibrating radio, from which emitted a most horrendous squalling noise. It appeared that some guy was in severe and terminal pain, and he was accompanied by what sounded like several drum, guitar and piano school flunkouts.

"What kind of garbage is that on the radio?" I asked, fighting back nausea.

"Aw, the new man coerced us into that," the older easygoing man replied. "He don't like country music."

"Do you reckon," I asked myself, "that those cows have their noses out of joint because they are forced to listen to some primitive animalistic-type rock music rather than country?" It seemed like I vaguely remembered reading somewhere of some researcher who had performed music trials with animals and certain melodious pieces were more conducive to contentment and production than others.

I decided to give it a try. I rotated the radio dial and quickly found George Jones soberly singing, "He Stopped Lovin' Her Today." As the milkers' eyes began to glaze over, the new man came into the parlor and looked over at me in astonishment.

"Hey, turn that back to the good music!" he screamed.

"Nothing doin'!" I retorted. "That rock music is giving these cows ulcers and making them nervous. The reason they won't come in to be milked is that they don't like your music."

"No, no!" he whined as he flung down a container of teat dip, "I can't stand that country junk!"

"Looka here, boy," I said firmly. "The health of these cows is my responsibility, and your loud rock music and your stick out yonder are the problems with production. I'd suggest that if you can't get with the program, perhaps you'd better get on the road."

By now his hands were shaking, his lips quivering and his eyes began to focus somewhere several miles behind where I was standing. I had seen rock music withdrawal symptoms before, in some of my students, and this guy was suffering from a severe case.

I met the owner coming in the door as I was going out.

"Well, what is it, Doc, what is it?" he nervously stammered between cigarette puffs.

"Very simple," I declared. "A classic case of rock music overload. You've either got to get shed of that new guy in there or get him to accept country music and quit traumatizing the cows."

"Aw, Doc, you can't be serious!"

"I'm serious as Sunday sin!" I replied. "If you'd spend more time in the parlor, and less time on the golf course, you'd see what was going on and wouldn't have to pay me a big consulting fee to tell you what you should already know. 'Course that's fine with me, 'cause consulting is a heap easier than paring out foot abscesses and pulling calves."

"O.K., O.K., I don't need no more of your classroom lecturing," he said with a frown. "Send me a bill. I'll take care of that rock music problem!"

As I drove off, Conway Twitty and Loretta Lynn were happily dueting a song about love and all the ramifications thereof. I pointed the truck in the general direction of the donut shop and wondered aloud.

"Maybe I'll start consulting just like some of my good friends. It might be lots of fun flying around all over the country, making sure the radios were all dialed to the proper country music station and running off all the guys with hoe-handle-type sticks!"

22

Fringe benefits of a farm veterinarian

OCCASIONALLY, when I meet nonfarm folks and they find that I am a livestock veterinarian, they often ask me, "Couldn't you make more money, and wouldn't it be easier work, if you just stayed in your office all day and doctored on dogs and cats?"

"Well, yes, I guess so, but that's not what I enjoy doing the most," is my usual reply.

Since they don't understand the workings of a farm, they wouldn't understand the feelings that my colleagues and I get in doing things that improve the health status of farm animals. There probably is no reason for them to understand the close relationship that develops over a period of time between a veterinarian and his or her farm family clients.

As far as making big money is concerned, no veterinarian is going to get rich in veterinary practice, in spite of the size of some of the vet bills you get. There are just too many drug bills and other expenses for vets to make a lot of money. Furthermore, I would do what I could to discourage prospective vet school applicants if I knew that they were looking for big dollars.

The most rewarding feature of being a veterinarian is being at the receiving end of the farm family generosity and good will. The feeling of jumping back into the truck after a tough calf delivery, and the umpteenth call that day, and finding a package of fresh sausage, some freshly picked snap beans, or some pear preserves on the seat, put there by some thoughtful family member, cannot be matched by money.

Visiting Harold Plocher's cherry trees and picking an OB sleeve full of ripe cherries is another fringe benefit. One word of caution here: Eating large amounts of fresh cherries at one sitting can be hazardous to your health. It is best to limit your fresh cherry intake to less than 2 percent of your body weight! The same precautions hold for watermelons, ice cream, fresh peaches, boiled peanuts and collard greens.

A visit to Claude's corn patch for some roast'n'ears (Southern for roasting ears) is always a treat, even if you go ahead and eat corn on the cob raw like one of my former employers used to do.

Few things are more enjoyable than mealtimes at a farmer's home. I have been privileged to park my feet under the best tables. For instance, we used to TB test the Dillon herd during the morning milking, before breakfast. As the sun came up, the entire family and Doc would be camped at a breakfast table that would make a king's table look pale and anemic. My partner and I argued over few things, but fighting over who got to go to that farm for TB testing was one of them.

I always liked to visit Brownie Alm's place in the middle of the morning if possible. That way I'd slip into his mama's kitchen and find that homemade bread she always had in the breadbox. I'd hack off a generous slab with the clean blade of my pocket knife and coat it with several gobs of genuine home-churned Jersey butter and munch on it while I sped to my next call. Usually, that would tide me over until dinner (that's Southern for lunch).

Stand in the creek . . .

At many dairies I have tried to time my visit or doctor on cows long enough that noontime caught me there. If it was dinnertime at Hobson Dubose's place, he'd twist my arm to stay and eat some of Mary's cooking. He didn't have to twist very hard because I knew that after the peas, fried chicken, cornbread, and other fixin's, she'd bring out a foot-tall, four-layered, diet-bustin' coconut cake. After that, I'd have to find a creek to stand in to keep from foundering.

Few mealtime sessions can compare with lunch at the Butlers, the Echols, the Hales, the Robinsons and dozens of others who sincerely enjoy feeding the Doc and his crew. You won't find this kind of fellowship and sincerity eating out at the "Big Burger."

When I was doing brucellosis testing on beef herds in Louisiana, noontime often caught me on some large ranch. If I played my cards right, the rancher would fix a big jambalaya for the workers. He would build a fire around a big iron pot and cook right near the corral. The only problem we ever had was when a particularly mean Brahman cow got between us and the pot, and the jambalaya stuck. We ate it burned anyway.

The Krauss farm was one of my favorite midafternoon calls. Mrs. Krauss put up the best dill pickles ever. She picked the cucumbers right out of her garden and used an old secret recipe that cannot be duplicated by anybody else. One day, she caught me in her pantry with dill pickles in both hands. So, the next time I was there she had 24 jars of those pickles for me all cased up and ready to go.

Now, the evening meal ought to be partaken at home or skipped. This is a time for families to be together and veterinarians shouldn't be eating supper with farmers, except in special situations. After-supper calls are another matter. Mighty high on the list would be a piece of Jessie Harrison's pecan, double rich, hunger-stompin' pie and a cup of her fresh coffee. A little conversation about the bulldogs and the corn crop and back on the road again.

These are the fringe benefits of working daily with farmers. I hope that The Master will allow me many more years of this type work. Since coming to work for the Veterinary College at Georgia, Drs. McDaniel, Blackmon and I try to teach students about the herd health concept. This puts us on a lot of dairy, beef, swine and sheep farms. There have been accusations from some of our less fortunate faculty colleagues that we limit our group visits to only those farms that serve outstanding meals. This is an absolute untruth! This is a slanderous rumor started by some jealous person who has to stay penned up in a stuffy office every day.

"Could I please have another piece of coconut cake, Mrs. Butler?"

23

"That's my best cow lyin' there"

THE herd consisted of 62 head of wild, unruly, Brahman-crossbred momma cows and their calves. I always dreaded working them, not only because they were so hard to handle, but also because it took so much time. Also, Mr. Jack Dempsey, the owner, never was present when we worked through them. This was bad in a way, since he never was around when certain decisions had to be made. But it also was good, since his hot temper could make things unpleasant.

This day we had worked 61 of them, but the last one was an old, mean, hard-core cow that refused to allow the farm workers to funnel her into the chute.

"Doc, could you 'hope' us with this here fool cow?" exclaimed Junior Jones. "We jus' can't git 'er to go in!"

It's always aggravating to lose time arguing with uncooperative cows. I find that it often is more expedient to lend a hand than to stand up in front of the chute yelling out various suggestions that usually don't work anyway.

One approach that occasionally works well on vicious cows is the "cow-chase-man" technique. It works like this. Some young, fleet-of-foot, gutsy person is selected as the sacrifice. He vaults into the pen with the beast, commences waving his arms wildly and shouting various insults and semiobscenities directly into the face of the cow.

If all goes as planned, the completely riled cow now lowers her head and charges the human offering, who turns and precedes the cow into the chute. A 2 by 6 scantling or a locust sapling is inserted crossways into the chute behind the beast but in front of two posts. The anxious chasee then vaults up over the side of the chute. Of course, the chasee should be careful not to stumble and fall, since that could be disastrous.

"Sure I'll help!" I yelled, as I bounded over the corral fence and commenced making faces at the cow. Seconds later, I was loping down the chute with the cow in close pursuit. I could feel her hot, snorty breathing on the back of my legs as I barely escaped up the chute side. She passed underneath me and crashed into the headgate as I hung on for dear life.

Crash! Bam! Clang! The chute rattled, shook and shuddered. Satch Johnson, the muscle-bound handyman, never had missed catching a cow in the old, worn-out Powder River chute, and today was no exception. The only problem was that she hit the gate head-on, kind of like a Mercedes running head-on into a road grader.

"Doc, her tongue's lolled out, but she ain't movin'! Her eyes done sot, too!" suddenly exclaimed Satch.

"Open the headgate" . . .

"Open the headgate! Open the headgate, quick!" I screamed as I jumped down from the six-foot corral fence.

I arrived up front presently, only to see Satch open the latch and the cow's head flop lifelessly out onto the ground. Her eyes were rolled up like she was looking at Saturn as she drew a final futile breath.

"Help me get 'er out of here, Satch," I yelled. We tugged and strained as the other workers came trotting up. Together we were able to drag her out of the chute and commence resuscitation efforts.

I never have had good luck bringing the dead back to life like they do every night on those hospital TV shows. After a few minutes of desperately pounding and jumping on her chest, it was obvious that she was not going to respond.

"It's no use, troops," I announced. "She broke her neck when she crashed into the headgate."

"Uh oh!" moaned Junior, "Mr. Dempsey, he ain't gon' lack this. He's gon' claim that this here was his best cow! He sez zat ever' time one of these idiots breaks her neck in this ol' piece of a chute."

"Yeah, that's right," replied Satch. "What you gon' tell 'im, Doc?"

They all stared at me expectantly, with lower jaws dropped and heads at a tilt.

"Wait a minute!" I exclaimed. "Why've I got to be the

one to call him. I didn't kill her! She just committed suicide! Wasn't my fault!"

They just stared at me, shaking their heads from side to side. Occasionally, they would look down at the deceased, cluck their tongues and make "tch, tch" noises, then stare back at me.

"Look! Mr. Dempsey's a'comin'!" mumbled Junior. "He's gonna be hot when he sees this!"

Sure enough, when we all straightened up and peered roadward, we saw the white, four-wheel-drive Ford as it barrelled down through the dried up pasture, barely outrunning a great cloud of beige-colored dust. About that time, the cowboy-hatted driver spied the quartet of workers looking down at the prostrate and very still figure of the bovine, and the vehicle seemed to speed up considerably.

Presently, the truck came sliding to a stop adjacent to the corral, and Mr. Dempsey alit from the driver's door in a rush. He and the dust cloud arrived cowside simultaneously.

"What is it, Doc? What's happening?" he coughed and stammered loudly as he gazed at the immobile figure on the ground. I noticed that he had a huge chew of tobacco in his right cheek.

"We ain't had nothin' to do wi' dis, Mr. Dempsey," pleaded Junior. "Doc done it. He made 'er go in 'ere an' she broke 'er neck!"

"What! Do somethin', John!" Mr. Dempsey screamed. "That's my best cow layin' there! Don't just stand there!"

"It's no use," I wheezed through the dust. "She's a goner. I reckon she hit that squeeze chute so hard that she broke her neck."

At that he ripped off his cheap straw cowboy hat and hurled it to the ground. Then he stomped it flat and began using terribly vile language. By now his face was the color of an Alabama football jersey.

"You can't have nothin'! You just can't have nothin'!" He then proceeded to attack the squeeze chute with swift side kicks of his size 12 leather boots. He picked up one of the locust saplings and broke it in half over the side of the poor, defenseless chute and then moved on back to the holding pen where he crushed a semirotten 2 by 10 with the

91

remaining stump of the sapling.

The other workers were scattering out of range of the fists, feet and flying saplings, but I just stood there, agape and agog. The closest thing I had seen to such a temper tantrum had been when a certain football coach made a fool of himself on national TV by abusing his players and any other objects within kicking range.

Suddenly, he stopped with broken sapling poised in mid-air and staggered up against my truck.

"He's havin' a spell," allowed Junior. "Look at how white his face's done got!"

"Oh, no!" I said to myself. "He's having a heart attack, and he's gonna die out here in this pasture!"

As he sank to the ground beside the truck, we eased over and started opening up his collar.

"What's the matter, Jack?" I finally heard myself say. After a pause of about five seconds, he finally spoke.

"Swallered my chaw," he whispered. "Git water! Quick!" Now he was coughing and gagging, trying to disgorge the great wad of tobacco that had slipped down his gullet. Within a few minutes, he was OK again but was somewhat subdued.

I learned two good lessons that day. First, working wild cattle is not without some risk to their well-being. Second, never get violently angry with a large chew of tobacco in your mouth. It would be a shame to lose both a man and a cow in the same cow-working episode.

24

"Doc, please wait just 30 more minutes"

I HAVE thought about it for a long time. Finally I have decided that, regardless of the time of the day or night that veterinarians close their clinics, someone either will come in after quitting time or will call and ask them to stay open a little longer.

About 11:30 one night, I was in the clinic checking on a poodle that I had operated on earlier in the day, when the phone rang.

"Doc, I've got this here dog that just scratches all the time. It's just drivin' us crazy! We can't sleep or nothin'! I wanta bring him over there and git you to give 'im one of them itch shots."

"Well, can't you come in tomorrow?" I asked. "I was just leaving."

"Doc, please wait just 30 more minutes," he begged. "I've got to go deer huntin' tomorrow, and my wife's car is broke down, so I got to bring him in tonight!"

So I waited. **After** he stopped by the Jiffy Mart and picked up a pack or two of "ready rolls," a liter of sugar water drench and jawed with the drunks that had stopped by on their way home from the state line, he leisurely motored on over to the animal clinic.

Mangy canine . . .

As I was heaving the mangy canine up onto the exam table, the phone rang again. This time it was dairyman I. C. Goodmilk honoring me with his annual call.

"Doc, I've got a fresh cow down, but I've run out of calcium. I just plum forgot to get a case the last time I was in the co-op. I need to run over there and borrow a couple jugs from you," he kind of ordered.

"O.K., I. C.," I said, "I'll be here."

"What's that thumpin' noise I hear, Doc?" I. C. queried, as the mutt in misery exhibited his world class scratching and thumping technique.

"Just a dog with fleas," I answered as I replaced the phone.

"He ain't got no fleas, Doc," my patient's owner retaliated haughtily. "I been puttin' dried cow manure on him and then keepin' pine shavin's in his bed. Unca Fred says . . ."

He couldn't finish because the phone went off right behind him. He jumped straight up.

"You still open, Doc?" the caller drawled, just as I death-gripped the phone and mashed my left ear with it.

"Naw, Sir," I said calmly, "we've closed up; thought we might try to get a few minutes of shut-eye before daylight."

"Well, I just thought I might run this gerbil over there and let you take a look at 'im, soon as the Johnny Carson show's over," he said thoughtfully. "This lil' ol' rat ain't been right for a month!"

"Why not!" I exclaimed. "Why don't you load up all the dogs, too, and we'll just bathe and dip 'em while you're here!" I hung up the phone gently and just stared at the wide-awake guy and his clawing canine.

"I'll swear! Why don't we just run outside, climb up to the top of the two-way tower and holler up everybody in the county! That way we'll save goin' through the middle man!" I said, in disbelief.

"Doc, you stay open pert near all night, don't you?" asked the mutt's owner, as he scanned the exam room wall, examining my diploma, licenses and awards from my FFA boys. The poor dog was scratching so hard now that the table was shaking like a seed cleaner, and hair and fleas were flying everywhere.

As I stared, a pickup truck came sliding to a stop in the gravel driveway in front of the clinic. I heard two doors slam, and two men were conversing.

"Aw, he won't care, Buck," one voice said. "He's here anyway!"

"Yeah, but it's so late," the other voice said. "Rover, let's go see if he'll clip your toenails an' give you a worm dose."

Just as Rover and friends got to the front door, two more vehicles turned in. One was I. C. after his calcium, and the other was the town's night policeman. He started shining his spotlight into the clinic and conversing over his loud-speaker.

"You O.K. in 'ere, Doc?" he blared loudly. "What's all those cars here for?"

Other cars were slowing down, pulling off onto the edge of the road; their occupants were getting out trying to see what was going on at the vet clinic, while others remained seated but were craning their necks in curious anticipation.

A transfer truck and Trailways bus both slowed down to a creep, and their drivers stared sleepily at the growing multitude. Brakes could be heard squealing, and clouds of dust were being raised as other cars ran off the road to avoid rear-ending others in the traffic jam.

When I finished with my flea-tormented patient in the exam room, I was greeted by a mass of humanity in the waiting area. Men were shaking hands with each other like they were long-lost buddies when, in reality, they had just seen each other hours ago when they left work together at the paper mill. Dogs were warily sniffing each other, and throaty growls were beginning to emit from their throats. A group of five or six men were over in the corner propped up on the stack of aureomycin crumbles telling Yankee jokes, while I. C. Goodmilk was exiting quickly with a case of calcium on his hip.

"Doc, I also got four dozen mastitis tubes and two liqua-mycins, too," he said. "Just charge it; maybe I can pay you one of these days!"

I just stood there momentarily, fuming. There I was, tired to the bone, with 400 cows to work in the a.m., and surrounded by a bunch of people who had nothing better to do than harass their vet at 1 o'clock in the morning. Then, suddenly, it hit me.

"What am I complaining about?" I said to myself. "These people all have legitimate needs and concerns or they wouldn't be here. They all feel comfortable with my work and my place of business or they wouldn't be here. And I'm making money. That's one reason why I'm here, and this doesn't happen that often."

With renewed vigor, I briskly strode over to the radio and dialed the all-night country music station. Roy Acuff was rendering out his "I Saw the Light" song. As more cars turned in outside, I waded into the crowd.

"Who's next?" I said cheerfully. "Let's get this work done and get home to bed!"

25

"It's a letter from the IRS, Dear"

I KNEW that it was going to happen sooner or later. So, when the very official looking, brown, windowed envelope arrived, I was not surprised to see "Internal Revenue Service, Mobile, Ala.," stamped in the upper left-hand corner.

That cold and tingly chill quickly ascended my spine as I ripped open the letter. I had felt the same chill before — like when I was "semigored" in the side by an enraged Brahman bull that I had tried to dehorn and again when I thought the baby had escaped.

"You are hereby notified . . ." the letter began. Why do these official letters always start out like that? Then it went on to say that I was being audited, and my presence would be required in their offices on such and such a date. I remember that the appointed date was on a Thursday.

"I can't go down there on Thursday," I raged. "Don't those idiots know that's sale barn day?"

"Now, Honey, just cool down," recommended Jan. "Getting yourself all riled up won't help anything. You'll just have to get someone to cover for you at the stockyard that day."

"There is no one else," I replied. "I'm the only one they've got!"

"John, when are you going to learn that you alone can't save the world? You simply cannot do everything by yourself and not ask for help from other people!"

"Maybe I'll call 'em and go in on a Saturday afternoon or night," I suggested.

"You know very well that government people don't go to the office on Saturday, or at night," she chided.

"Well, I can't worry with it right now," I said, hurriedly. "I've got to go test those cows up at the Norman Lewis place."

I fled the office and kangarooed into the driver's seat of my truck. As I yanked the handle into "drive" and goosed the accelerator, my rage continued.

"Those idiots!" I fumed to myself. "Here I am barely making ends meet by pulling calves, getting kicked and stomped by bulls and mules and wading through mud and manure. Now they want to audit me because they don't have sense enough to understand the real world! I wish that whole crowd would follow me around for just one day!"

A few minutes later I realized that I was leaning over the steering wheel, my teeth were gritting and the truck literally was rocketing down the roadway since my foot had the accelerator smashed flat on the floorboard. I was passing slower vehicles like they were standing still, and my backwash was blowing hats and caps off pedestrians, as well as scaring them witless.

People who were sweeping their yards and picking okra in their roadside gardens were stopping in the midst of their labors to stare at the speeding white truck with its two-way radio antenna laid back almost parallel to the truck body.

Moments later, I turned off the main highway onto Indian Creek Road — a narrow, clay-based trail. Great clouds of dust and flying gravel were left in the wake of my forward progress. Suddenly, as I crested a small hill, there was Goat, the mailman. He was also traveling much too fast for the one-lane road. In addition, he had his eyes focused downward into the front seat, still sorting his cards and letters. I felt that cold chill again.

Hit the ditch . . .

The only way to avoid a head-on collision was to hit the ditch and take my chances.

"Wham! Bam! Crunch! Scrape! Pow!" uttered the truck as metal was greeted rudely by rocks, dirt, saplings and dead limbs. It's always shocking how loud a collision can be.

Luckily, I had missed Goat, mainly because he had seen me at the last moment, and he, too, had hit the ditch on his side.

Momentarily, we both just sat in our vehicles, stunned

and shocked over the fast-paced event of the past three seconds. Finally, doors cracked open, and the two shaking occupants emerged from the ditched truck and car. Both vehicles were mired in the wet ditch and were slanted at almost 45-degree angles.

"Goat," I said, as I brushed dust off my pants, "we got to stop meetin' like this."

"D-D-Doc!" he stammered, "you scare-scare-scared me to d-d-death!" Goat had a tendency to stutter when he got excited. "We-we nearly hit h-h-head on!"

"Yeah, neither one of us were payin' attention to business," I said. "Look, I'll call Jan on the radio, and she can call Johnny over at the Norman Lewis place. He'll come and pull us out with that WD-45."

Truck and car damage were minor. My truck had received the worst end of it. The right door was scraped, but it already was dented in, compliments of a wild yearling on the end of a rope. The right front light was smashed out, and the bumper was pushed back into the fender.

Goat and I sat down on the kudzued ditch bank and conversed while Johnny was on his way.

"Goat, you ever been audited by the IRS?"

"Naw, Doc," he answered, "b-b-but two of my brothers have."

"Well, can you change the date of the audit? They want me to come in on sale barn day."

"Yeah, I think you can. I know when they g-g-got Jack, he had to be in court the same day, so they just came to his office and did it there."

That sounded good. I figured if they were on my home field rather than me being on theirs, I would have a definite advantage. I felt better already! There wasn't any reason to panic, since the IRS people were just doing their job, and surely they meant no harm. After all, I wasn't a criminal! I had done nothing wrong!

Out of the ditch . . .

Finally, Johnny came and extracted both Goat and me from the ditches. I completed the work at the Norman Lewis place and headed back to the clinic to make the phone call to the IRS.

"Good afternoon, Internal Revenue Service," a honey-sweet-voiced Southern belle answered when the call finally got through. "May I help you?"

How nice she was! Someone that pleasant surely had no malice in her heart towards a poor, hard-working tax-payer.

I briefly told her my problem, and she seemed sincerely interested in trying to help.

"Sir, let me connect you with Agent Jones. He has been assigned as your primary auditor."

Within seconds, a gruff, no-nonsense man was curtly barking over the phone. He sounded like a Marine sergeant.

"This is Agent Jones speaking. What is the problem?"

"Well, you have my audit scheduled for Thursday. That's by far my busiest day and . . ."

"Why so busy on Thursday?" he quickly queried.

"I'm the veterinarian in charge at a stockyard, and I have to be present for testing and vaccinating cattle and swine. I've got to be there every Thursday. Do you reckon you could make it another day of the week? Also, could you come to my office?"

There was a lengthy pause on the far end of the phone line. I could hear the shuffling of paper and flipping of calendar pages.

"This is somewhat irregular, Mr. McCormack," he ordered, "since I seldom perform on-site audits, except in special hardship cases."

I spent the next few moments trying to convince him of why he should come to my office. Finally, he spoke.

"Actually, I do have to be in your community two weeks from Tuesday to seize some property from a delinquent taxpayer. I'll just come by your place then. I'll spend the night and finish your books the next day.

I gulped hard when he said the word "seize." He seemed to relish saying it so much.

"Yessir, Agent Jones," I said weakly, "that will be just fine."

"Oh, by the way, Mr. McCormack," he asked, "please tell me — do you have to go to school in order to be a veterinarian . . .?"

I felt the cold chill again . . .

100

26

The IRS, Part II

WHEN the day of the big IRS audit arrived, I arose early from a nightmarish sleep and proceeded to the clinic. After looking in on the small animal patients in the kennel room, I went into the storage room, moved supplies and drugs around and created a clean spot for the agent. I then set up a card table and chair where he could work undisturbed. I figured that he would be impressed with my thoughtfulness and would have mercy on me when he was checking the books.

I didn't know what time Mr. Jones would arrive since I was to be his second victim that day. His first one was to be minus his property by the time the agent arrived at my clinic. I was afraid that he would be in a rank mood when he got to me, so I found some fake flowers and made an "oleo" bouquet and set it on the desk. In addition, I piled all the income tax returns that he had requested, all my record books and day books, pencils and pads and an adding machine neatly beside the flowers. Surely my efficiency and the nice flowers would make points with a dedicated federal servant.

At 11:25 a.m., I saw the new, plain, black Ford turn slowly into the clinic parking lot. Through the exam room window I saw the agent look at his watch, then at his odometer and carefully make an entry into a plain, gray ledger book. Next, he rolled up the window on the driver's side, opened the door, got out and locked all the doors.

"Wow, what a weirdo he must be," I thought to myself, since no one ever locked their truck around home, many not even their houses. At the time, there was no need to do such a thing.

From the trunk he retrieved an old, well-used, dark gray briefcase, two large manila folders and an ancient adding machine. When he started for the front door, I got there first, opened it up and stood there grinning.

"Yes, Sir!" I beamed, "Good morning, good morning! You must be Agent Jones. Come right on in this house!"

"Mr. McCormack, I presume," he announced in a very business-like manner. "Yes, I'm Agent T. K. Jones, and I'm here to investigate your tax irregularity. Would you direct me to your business office?"

"Well, I don't reckon I have a business office," I countered, "but I have fixed you up a nice, quiet place in the storage room."

I led him down the hall and into the spare room that was nearly full of junk, drugs and other clinic supplies.

"How's this?" I asked proudly. "You won't be disturbed here with barking dogs and people going and coming."

"Well," he said as he looked around suspiciously, "this is somewhat irregular, but I suppose I can make do with these meager facilities. I see that you have all your records right here. Good!"

"Is there anything I can get for you?" I asked. "I do have a right smart of work ahead of me."

What's that smell?

"No, I think not, but don't vacate the area since it may be necessary to interrogate you at length about some of these records," he ordered. "By the way, what is that pungent odor?"

I sniffed the air several times but didn't catch anything unusual, so I just shook my head from side to side.

"It seems to be coming from the vicinity of those sacks over there," he said, as he pointed into the corner.

"Oh yeah, that's just some aureomycin crumbles right there. That drum in the corner has mineral oil in it, and those buckets contain horse vitamins. That's probably what you are smelling. I just love that smell, don't you?"

He just stared at me with his nose wrinkled up. I gathered that he didn't like the unique smell of a vet clinic.

"Bet you've been to a lot of animal clinics over the years, haven't you?" I asked, trying hard to be neighborly, as well as change the subject.

"Negative, this is my initial case," he replied, as he rearranged the desk to suit his own tastes. It appeared that he was going to stay for a pretty good spell.

"But you have checked veterinarians before," I pleaded.

"Negative, you're the first and only."

I felt that same cold chill shooting up my spine again. I was hoping that he would know something about the nature of my work so we could converse intelligently.

At noon, he went back out to his car with briefcase in hand and ate his lunch in the front seat. I offered him cheese, bologna, bread and an RC cola from the clinic refrigerator, but he declined with a great show of refusal. I believe he thought that I was trying to bribe him with cold cuts.

While he lunched, I left and made several farm calls. I tried not to worry about the strange man back at my office, but I couldn't help it. I kept having horrible visions of me being handcuffed and carted off to the jailhouse. Then I would shake my head to clear it of those insane thoughts.

"Base to unit one, base to unit one. Do you read?" It was Jan on the two-way.

"Yeah, come on base."

"John, the tax man wants to ask you some questions about the records. I'm going to put him on."

"OK." I noticed that I was white-knuckling the steering wheel and getting heavier on the accelerator.

"Uh, Mr. McCormack," Mr. Jones' voice carried over the airways. "There are some odd entries in your record books and receipts that I need to ask you about. First of all, here is where you allegedly paid $120.50 for a calf named Jack. Would you please explain."

"Mr. Jones, I don't know what you're talking about. Just hold tight and I'll be there shortly. I can't converse very well with you over this radio."

As I beelined homeward, I tried hard to recollect buying a calf. I was certain that I had not made any such purchase in the years for which I was being audited. I did remember breaking a calf's foreleg once while trying to deliver it with a calf jack, and the owner gave me the calf.

Then it hit me! Calf jack! Of course! I had bought a calf jack, and he just didn't understand the veterinary jargon.

"It's not a calf named Jack," I yelled as I charged through the clinic door. "It's a calf jack."

"What's a calf jack?" asked the puzzled fed.

"We use a calf jack to assist a cow in labor. When used properly, the jack pulls on the calf to complete the delivery," I relayed.

"All right, that's a sufficient explanation," he replied. "Now I have a few other questions. What is the use of a squeeze chute?"

After I convinced him of the necessity of a squeeze chute, he asked about several other items. He wanted to know why my gasoline bill was so outrageous, wanted an explanation of my high drug bills and even questioned the one vet meeting I had attended the previous year.

Two hours later, and much more knowledgeable about veterinary medicine, Mr. Jones packed up his gear and started out.

"It has been a pleasure, Doctor," he smiled. "I admire greatly the work that you are doing for the animal kingdom. You surely opened my eyes about your profession. Sorry about addressing you as 'Mister.'"

"Well, that's good," I replied. "When will I know the results of your audit?"

"In about two weeks you will receive a report," he said. Then he got into his plain car, made an entry in his book and slowly pulled away from the clinic. I never saw him again.

I felt good about the audit until the letter arrived three weeks later. When I read it, I had cold spinal chills, hot flashes and a fainting spell. The biggest problem was improper depreciation of a calf jack, squeeze chute and two trucks. In addition, there were several other violations, and they demanded their money immediately. I remember clearly that the bill was the equivalent of 125 calf deliveries. That's a pretty steep price to pay just to be called "Doctor."

27

Carney Sam's thoughts on the moon walk

IT WAS a hot, muggy morning in late July, as I hustled around dead man's curve. Down the road I could make out Mrs. Ruby McCord's general store shining in the bright sunlight.

My stomach was ready for a milk medication break, since it had been aching more than usual that morning. Maybe it was the hassle of bleeding 400 head at the stockyard the day before, or perhaps it was the two C-sections I had done alone the night before.

This day the phone had awakened me before daylight with more emergencies, most of which should have been taken care of the day before. I just had too much work to do and not enough time to get it done. I was tired, half sick, cranky and my ulcer was burning. Therefore, Miss Ruby's simple little country store was like an oasis in the desert to me. It offered a few minutes' rest where I could numb my stomach pain with her cold sweet milk and exchange conversation with friends.

The store was just perfect for the area. It had one old Sinclair gas pump where a handle had to be rocked back and forth in order to get the gasoline up into the glass container at the top. There was a large Royal Crown Cola sign nailed up at the gable that read, "McCord's Groc. & Ser. Sta." In the South everything is shortened. Chicken mash in flowery sacks was piled outside the front door, and four cats dove underneath the building as I jumped from the truck in a run.

This day it appeared that Miss Ruby had two guests. A wagon and team of mules were tied to a magnolia tree, and an old pickup truck with both doors missing was backed up to the side of the store as if it were ready in case a quick getaway was necessary. The truck belonged to Carney

Sam Jenkins, local homemade veterinarian, natural-born philosopher and gifted seer. The team belonged to his understudy, Buck Tutt.

"Doc, derned if you don't look like you been rode hard an' put up wet!" barked Carney Sam. "What'd you do last night?"

I strode quickly toward the old refrigerator and robbed it of a quart of Borden's. As I drenched myself with it, I could feel almost immediate relief as it sloshed over my irritated gastric mucosa.

"Somethin' for ya, Doctuh?" Miss Ruby said. She always said that, but she always expected me to go get it myself.

"Jus' he'p yo'se'f."

Carney Sam and Buck both were sitting on nail kegs, drinking R.C. colas, eating moon pies and firing questions at me.

"Just shut up a minute, Carney Sam," I exploded. "Gimme a chance to get my breath. I didn't come in here to take another state board exam!"

"Well, jus' lissen to 'im, Buck, ain't he somethin' this mornin'! He sho is talkin' mighty smart alecky to 'is friends!"

"Yeah," chimed in Buck, "jus' 'scuse us, Mr. Doctuh! You kin jus' git offen yo' high hoss an' quit insultin' everbody!"

"Alright," I apologized, "I'm sorry. I'm just tired, wore out from working all night and I hurt all over."

"By the way," I said, trying to change the subject, "did y'all see those astronauts walk on the moon this mornin'? Wasn't that somethin'!"

"Doc, are you serious?" replied Carney Sam, as he looked around at an agreeing Buck. "You don't really believe that actually happened, do you?"

"Sure I believe it. I saw it on TV at the hardware store!"

Filmed in "Arizoner" . . .

"It's lies! All lies!" he said, in disbelief at my ignorance. "It's all a put-up job, jus' to git mo' money. What they done, was to go way out yonder to Arizoner or Orgun where there's plenty of desert and wasteland and take all them TV pitchers there."

106

"Aw, come off it, Carney!" I declared, open mouthed, "You know the government wouldn't be a party to anything like that!"

"Doc, all this space and moon walkin' bizness ain't nothin' more than a deliberately planned plot by the gov'mint. They'll show some guys in funny suits walkin' on a stage that's made up to look like the moon. Folks that don't know no better will get all excited about it. Then Washington will raise taxes, collect a few more millions and them politicians will line their pockets with more and more of our hard-earned dollars.

"Tell you what, Doc," Carney Sam stated, "see if yo' income taxes ain't a whole lot higher nex' year. They'll go up more every year, too, every time they show one of them rockets blastin' off on TV. Just wait and see!"

"Look," I said, as I backed towards the door. "I don't have time to stand here and argue with a couple of 19th century dwellers who haven't got enough sense to accept reality. I've got to go put a prolapse back in."

As I went out the door, I could hear Buck as he echoed what Carney Sam had just said.

"Doc, you'll see, you'll see!"

I hurried to my next call while pondering the asinine theory that I had just heard. As I became immersed in the day's activities though, I soon forgot about the space program.

Several farmers did comment about how wasteful it was.

"They shoulda' took some of that money and put a bridge over Puss Cuss Creek or somethin' useful like that," commented L. Z. Watson. "We have to ford that creek every time we go to town. And when the water gits high, we are cut off."

"It's a funny thing to me," complained Bo Jack Murphy, "how the gov'mint can shoot millions of dollars up to the moon, but they won't give me but $25 a head for gittin' shed of these here Bang cows. All that space stuff is for is to give a bunch of them scientists and politicians soft jobs!"

When I arrived home that night, Tom, my oldest son, was out in the yard scanning the dark skies with my old binoculars.

"Whatcha doin', hoss fly?" I asked as I detrucked.

"Aw, I'm just looking up at the moon trying to see if there are any signs of life up there."

"Well, do you see anything?"

"Can't tell, Daddy," he replied. "If there's any sign of those astronauts, I don't see it."

"Do you have some doubts?" I asked.

"Well, I guess not," he said slowly, "but Junior Jenkins and Bo Tutt both claimed at school today that it was all fake and that what we saw on TV actually was filmed out on a desert in Arizona."

"That's odd," I replied, "I heard the same thing today, too. 'Course, it was from those guys' daddies."

Later on that night, I slipped out with the binoculars and looked up at the moon. I didn't see any dust up there, nor any other signs of men or machines. Do you reckon Carney Sam had been right? He did have a reputation for always having the right answers.

I do know this. My taxes went up a lot that year, and have increased every year since then. I just wonder . . .

28

The last cob fight

IN THIS day of television, computer games and loud stereo music, our offspring are missing out on one of nature's most challenging and competitive contests. An event that requires certain skills in selecting proper ammunition, considerable advance thought in maneuvering one's self into adequate hiding places, an accurate but restrained throwing arm and exceptionally adept footwork, since this pastime takes place entirely within the confines of the barnyard.

I am referring to that age-old game that once was played wherever corn was grown and hogs slopped and fed, the cob fight.

Back in the good old days of the 1940's, there wasn't much to do when relatives gathered together after church on Sunday afternoon. After as much of the bountiful meal could be eaten as possible, all the menfolk retired to the front porch or sitting room, depending on the season, and discussed with much authority such things as crops, politics, government interference and local events.

When it was decided that everyone could stand unaided on unfoundered feet and walk comfortably without causing serious weight damage to the ground, the routine trek to the barn and other outbuildings began. Since all present were farmers, each was interested in everyone else's past accomplishments and future plans. Last year's failures were not discussed much.

The cows were observed, fat pigs admired, hay sniffed, silage fondled, a few ears of corn shucked, tobacco examined and a host of other farm commodities discussed, approved and criticized. Eventually, the men would start easing on back towards the house, kicking clods and nibbling on straws while they made profound announcements and bragged about what they were going to do "next year."

By this time, some of the younger folk, especially the boys, had begun to lag behind the procession and get into devilment, as Pa would say.

"Cob fight!" yelled Cousin Carl one Sunday afternoon. All the kids scattered to get ammunition.

Now Carl was the usual instigator of such activity. Today, he would have been called "hyperactive." Back then he was said to be "full of meanness." He and I always were on opposite sides in any contest. He was stronger, better looking, had a better arm, could kick a football farther, could run faster and grow more corn than I could. To make matters worse, he always was first to go barefooted in the springtime. I did have one advantage over Carl — I was smarter and made better grades. Strangely enough, that did help in a cob fight, since I usually could outwit him.

As we all scattered like quail, I turned to investigate his position. A cob whirred dangerously close to my forehead as I saw Carl streaking for the barn. Running for the cover of two empty Borden milk cans, I quickly planned my next moves. I would ease along the rail fence, hide briefly behind the water trough, then in a crouching position, sprint to the back of the hog house, climb over the fence and fill my pockets with the hard, weathered, mud caked corncobs. The other participants in the contest already were making their breaks to the hog lot for the same purpose.

Cob selection . . .

There was an art in selecting the proper type cobs. The secret was to find those that had been lying and aging in the hog lot for about a year, were dark brown to black in color, were hard and about three to four inches in length. Fresh cobs, especially white ones, were totally worthless for throwing since they were too light, wouldn't carry well or hold a good line.

Long ones wouldn't fit between thumb and forefinger, so they couldn't be thrown with any degree of accuracy. You usually had to throw long ones like a boomerang. If the cobs had been in the lot too long, they became like slivers of petrified wood that could open up long gashes in opponents' faces and backs of heads. Therefore, for humane

110

reasons, good judgment was called for when making your selections.

I knew that Carl would be in the barn loft because from there, he could hold his attackers at bay and hide amongst the hundreds of hay bales stored there.

Creeping out of the hog lot into the shadow of the big barn, I heard him jump from a bale of hay onto the loft floor. Looking up, I saw the side of his head appear at a hole where a board had fallen. For some reason I immediately let fly with my best throwing cob, even though head shots were strictly illegal.

"Spppllatt!"

It was a perfect shot that caught him on both his left ear and that little hard spot right behind the ear. You could even see the little rooster tail that sprung up from his perfectly slicked down, coal black hair. With blood dripping and him screaming at the top of his lungs, he sprinted towards the loft ladder to surrender and go tell on whoever had wounded him.

After about six steps, I heard a board-popping crash, another even higher pitched wail and a loud commotion in a horse stall. In his hasty retreat, Carl had stepped on a rotten board and fallen into the middle of the stall with old Nell, one of our gray mares. Nell was going berserk, trying to kick herself out of the stall and attempting to climb over the partition into the stall with Belle, her running mate. In the meantime, Carl, wide-eyed, was trying to avoid Nell's flying hooves and crawl to safety.

Was as good as dead . . .

When I finally realized the gravity of the situation, I panicked and ran to the back of the barn, stepped in a huge mud hole and fell in. Not only did I have on my "Sunday only" slippers, I also had on my new suit pants. Oh no, I was dead! Poor old Carl, he was just wounded with a long but shallow laceration to his hard head, probably a sore behind and maybe even stomped severely by an enraged and totally ignorant equine. But I was as good as dead for ruining my clothes!

Unknown to Carl and me, some of the girls had seen and heard the unfortunate events and had made a beeline to the house to announce loudly to the grownups that Carl and

John had half killed each other at the barn and their new clothes were in rags. This report sent parents of all descriptions bursting through all available exits of the house. Mothers were wiping their hands on aprons, and Pappas, with nostrils flared, were going at a half trot.

When the massive parent delegation arrived at the barn, Carl and I were standing side by side in the big hallway, using corn shucks to wipe the mud off our clothes. We looked like two horrible hallucinations. Blood and mud covered, we knew for sure that judgment day was at hand.

At that point, tight-lipped parents started cutting peach tree switches 10 feet long and as big around as hoe handles, ripping slick leather belts out of their britches, producing paddles with holes bored in them. I'm sure I even saw one fuming father jerk an electric chair out of the trunk of a 1937 Ford. The next few minutes are somewhat blurred in my memory, but each time I try to remember the exact happening, I get a severe pain to the rear and several inches below my belt.

Needless to say, when our appetites finally returned several days later, Carl and I ate several meals while standing. Thus ended a long series of championship cob fights. I am thankful, however, that the games were terminated before serious injury occurred.

Do you suppose that our country would be better off today if swift punishment was carried out by our court system the way our parents did back then? I do know this. I haven't chunked any more corncobs at anyone lately, and furthermore, I have absolutely no desire to do so!

29

News of my big mistake spread quickly

Have you got her penned up?" I asked loudly over the static on the phone line.

"Why she's just a plum pet, Doc," the barely audible voice on the other end of the long distance line replied. "We won't have no trouble at all ketchin 'er."

The call had come in from the adjoining county to the east. The caller, a Mr. Buckie Lee Davis, had brought his coon dogs over to my office on previous occasions, but I never had visited his backwoodsy farm for the purpose of treating his large animals.

This day his complaint was an old cow that was lame in the left rear leg. According to him, the cow was moaning, groaning, and grimacing with severe pain when she even considered the idea of moving. Buckie Lee was so emphatic in insisting that she was practically immobile that I didn't even try to convince him of the need for getting her restrained or penned. That was my first mistake.

While driving over to see Buckie Lee's cow, I thought about him, his name and his life-style.

"What a great name — Buckie Lee," I thought to myself.

When I was much younger, I often had wished that my name had been "Buck." It was such a tough sounding name. To me, it presented an image of a tanned and muscular individual who stood for the best in rugged and independent country living. A "Buck" type always drove a new four-wheel-drive pickup truck, with two weapon-filled gun racks over the rear window.

Buckie Lee's daddy had named him at birth, and his mama had added the "ie" on the end of the Buck. Somehow, he never had shed the boyhood handle of "Buckie," even though he now was six feet two and weighed about 210 pounds. He made good money by working the graveyard shift at the paper mill and farmed in the daytime.

My appearance at his driveway gate was announced by the penned coon hounds. I could see them leaping up onto their kennel fence beside the garage, throwing their heads back and barking with great enthusiasm.

Buckie Lee bounded down the back porch steps, threw a quick grimace toward the dog pen, which resulted in instant tail-tucked silence, and presented himself at truckside.

"Hey, Doc," he smiled, "thanks for coming. She's down under the hill behind the barn."

"Can we drive to where she is?"

"Sure. I'll just get in and ride."

That was our second mistake. I have found since that "plum pets" do not like strange vehicles invading their territory. That goes double for vet trucks that are white and have aerials.

As we approached the patient, she slowly raised her head from her midmorning grazing and warily peered at the unknown vehicle. She was holding that left rear leg about six inches off the ground and made no move to bear weight on it.

"Why don't you take that rope on the floorboard and lay it on her head," I said to Buckie Lee.

He immediately detrucked with lariat hidden behind his back and walked slowly toward the old overweight, brindle shorthorn cow. After several kind remarks uttered in a soothing tone, Buckie Lee gingerly looped the rope over her head.

"Make a halter with it, Buckie, so we can hold her better if she decides to run."

"Aw I got 'er now, Doc," he grinned, "she ain't goin' nowhere."

That was my third mistake.

I hopped from the truck and headed for that left rear foot. The instant I touched her she bellowed and started to sprint.

"Hold on, Buckie, hold on!" I pleaded.

Buckie Lee was holding on with all his might. With the end of the lariat wound crazily around his right arm, he didn't have any other choice. For a while he was matching the cow's pace, stride for stride, until the tip of his toe caught the corner of a pine stump.

Suddenly, Buckie Lee appeared to do a well-executed, but unintentional, belly flop onto the soggy lowlands. With the rope still knotted around his arm, he became a human sled as the wildly loping and bellowing bovine seemed to gather speed, even though she was motoring on three legs.

"Turn 'er aloose, turn 'er aloose!" I yelled loudly.

However, my shouting had no effect since the splashing noises created by Buckie Lee's skidding carcass and the oral vocalization of the cow prevented it.

Poor old Buckie Lee. No telling how much mud and grass had been scooped up by the front of his trousers as his front side furrowed a deep rut in the muddy lowlands. Nevertheless, he hung on with bulldog tenacity until the cow finally became exhausted about 100 yards away.

I had been trying to keep up with the cow-man duo, with black bag in hand, in hopes that I could get to the rope and end the chaos. Now, I saw my chance.

"Hang on, Buckie," I pleaded, "and I'll give her a shot of this penicillin. I reckon she's just got the foot rot."

That was my fourth mistake.

I injected the worn-out cow without picking up and examining the sore foot. Buckie Lee was not hurt, other than a few dozen scratches, a sore belly and ruined trousers.

My pride was injured, though, two weeks later when Carney Sam Jenkins pulled a roofing nail out of that foot. The news of my big mistake spread quickly and thoroughly throughout the three counties in which I worked. It became so bad that for awhile, I couldn't even stop at any of my favorite country stores for Vienna sausages and soda crackers without the proprietor or some store sitter bringing up Buckie Lee's cow and that infernal roofing nail in her foot.

I learned three very valuable lessons from that case. First, I now aggressively insist that all pet cows be haltered and tied or corralled before I arrive. Second, I always look at the bottom of sore feet, as well as the top. You won't miss seeing nails imbedded in the sole that way. Third, avoid stopping at country stores in the area after you've made a mistake at a nearby farm — unless you enjoy being constantly reminded of your error.

30

Half price for half a calf

W HEN I was a student in veterinary school many years ago, most of my professors did a fine job of teaching my classmates and me how to vaccinate animals properly, deliver a calf, take out a corn, or trim a set of ears on a Boxer dog. They even tried to teach us ethical behavior and how to hold a teacup with that little finger stuck out just right so we'd be socially acceptable. That didn't take with some of my classmates, however.

I do wish, though, that they had given us more lectures on business and how to run the financial end of a practice. Today, we still send our graduates out into the world with very little information along that line, so most are financial amateurs.

"About this here bill, Doc," a farmer drawled one morning, while I was restocking my truck for the day.

"Well, what about it?" I asked, as he handed me the document.

"It's just too high, Doc; I can't pay that much," he said, as if in real bad pain. "The pig died anyway, even after all them shots you give 'im! Can't you knock a little off on account of him dyin'?"

It's always been hard for me to explain to people that, just because the patient died, my drugs, supplies and vehicle costs don't suddenly stop. Whether the goat lives or dies, I still have the same amount of cash gone forever out of my own pocket. Therefore, I always have tried to charge a fair fee, and I don't believe in negotiating over a charge.

I called a lady once about a four-month-old overdue bill on a horse that I had dewormed and given its spring vaccinations.

"Oh, I meant to pay that," she apologized, "but last week that poor horse got struck by lightning out there in the pasture. Do I still have to pay even if he's dead?"

"I think it's only right for you to settle your account, ma'am, since the work I did for you was such a long time ago."

"Well, okay, I'll pay you anyway, but I don't see why I should have to," she lamented.

When the check came, down at the bottom left it said, "For — dead horse." It really burns me up for someone to write that on a check.

"Send me a bill, Doc, if I owe you anything," is another saying commonly uttered by farmers. One of my so-called friends uses this phrase a lot.

We will have visited his farm and vaccinated 300 head for lepto, dehorned 30 calves, opened up four-foot abscesses, cleaned off two cows that calved a week ago and left a gross of mastitis tubes. As I crawl weakly back to the truck with tongue lolled out and covered with every imaginable type cow excretion, secretion and discharge, I always will hear Paul's voice.

"Send me a bill, Doc, if I owe you anything!"

Some people want to pay half price for delivering half a calf. Simple Simon Tucker, a rancher near the salebarn where I worked on Thursdays, trucked in a half Charolais heifer one day many years ago. She was trying to deliver the rear half of a 100-pound-plus three-quarter Charolais fetus. The front half had been extracted sometime in the previous 24 hours with the aid of a 6N Ford tractor, several cowboys and pouches of chewing tobacco.

After about an hour's worth of grunting, straining and groaning on my part, I was able to get some embryotomy wire into the birth canal and looped over in between the calf's rear legs. Then with a sawing motion, I was able to split the pelvis in half. Next, I turned each hind quarter around and extracted them individually but not without a fair amount of tugging and straining.

As I stood there quivering with complete exhaustion and with not a clean spot on my coveralls, Simple Simon asked "The question."

"Owe ye anything?"

"Bout $20, I reckon," I said in a weak whisper.

"$20!" he screamed. "That's the regular price for pulling a whole calf! Heah, Doc, you take this $10 and go on."

All of a sudden, I wasn't weak anymore. It is amazing what sudden rage will do for weak muscles sometimes. I remember lunging for his throat and wiping my foul-smelling hands on the front of his bib overalls. I also remember he paid the full price and did not want a receipt. Sometimes you have to fight fire with fire. This approach may not work with every nonpaying customer, however.

Here are some favorite quotations from clients of mine in the years past, regarding their vet bills.

"Doc, I don't mind paying for your new clinic, new truck and that new X-ray machine," a farmer friend chided one day, "but I didn't want to pay it all this month!"

"Doc, you charge as much as a real doctor!"

"He may not know much about sick hogs, but he sure does know how to charge!"

"One of them stalls oughta have my name on it. I done paid for it twice!"

"Why don't you just come on out here and load up the cows and take 'em for the bill, Doc. They're not worth that much."

"Doc's the only vet I know of who's got a cash register on the front seat of his truck."

My favorite and most common comment was made by one John L. Doe. I vaccinated a drove of hogs for him one day, fixed several ruptured pigs and sold him some mange spray. As requested, I sent him a bill. And another, and another, and another. Finally, I went out to see him about the delinquent account after scribbling threatening notes on the last two bills.

He invited me into the house and Mrs. Doe fed us on coffee and homemade fruitcake. After 30 minutes, he never had mentioned the account, so I figured I would.

"John L.," I said carefully, "I sure do need to collect on that vet bill you owe me."

"What bill?" he asked, his forehead furrowed in wonder. He scratched his head and squenched up his eyes as if in deep thought. That's when I realized that some people never read the mail and also have very short memories.

I'll bet all veterinary practices have one of these jokers on their books.

118

31

"Dixie isn't gonna make it"

It WAS a few minutes before midnight on New Year's Eve at the VFW dance hall. Jan and I were having a great time dancing to an old-time band that specialized in Glenn Miller tunes.

As we cavorted about on the dance floor with our friends, I heard a familiar voice call my name from the vicinity of the front door.

"Oh no!" I said to Jan, "that's Carney Sam Jenkins over there behind me, isn't it?"

"Yep, sure is," she said with a sigh. "Why don't you go hide behind the piano?"

It was too late. He had spied me in the semidarkness and was shuffling our way. As usual, he had on his engineer's boots, red checkered flannel shirt and Funk's G hybrid cap.

"Carney Sam!" I exclaimed. "What are you doin' here, Boy? I didn't know you were a dancer!"

"Evenin', Doc. How're you, Miz Doc," he said as he ripped off his cap in respect to the lady present. He always called Jan "Miz Doc."

"Doc, Werner Fred — that's my boy, you know — his ole mare, the one we call Dixie, is doin' poorly. I've been foolin' with 'er near 'bout all night, but I just can't get her to respond. She's a hurtin'!"

"Has she got the colic?" I asked as he followed Jan and me as we waltzed around the floor.

"Yeah, Doc, 'at's right. I've drenched her with chinaberry tea, turpentine, coal oil, and I've even tried mine and yo' Choctaw County Colic Cocktail that we mixed up that night at Miss Ruby's place."

Jan was beginning to drum her fingers on my shoulder and her lips were beginning to purse, which indicated growing impatience with Carney Sam, as well as with me. She didn't much like him anyway, since he never called for help except late at night or on Sundays or holidays. Also, she didn't like it that he was a homemade vet who didn't have to pass state board exams, pay license fees or take out malpractice insurance.

At present though, people were staring at the three of us as we glided around the dance hall, trying to talk above the sounds of the orchestra.

"Look, let's go over yonder in the corner and have a glass of punch and decide what we're gonna do," I said finally.

Jan was really peeved now. She knew that I probably would go out to Carney Sam's old rocky hillside farm and spend the rest of the night there sitting up with that mare.

While Carney Sam and I sipped on our punch, Jan joined some of her cohorts and left us to discuss the sick mare.

It seemed that Werner Fred and Tootie Turner had taken Carney Sam's old pickup truck over into the next county and purchased a load of alfalfa hay. The mare had feasted on the new hay which was considerably higher in protein and energy than the old fescue and bermuda that she had been used to. Now she had a bad case of colic that was causing her much distress.

"I've got to go see about Werner Fred's horse," I told Jan, "you can ride home with Loren and Geraldine. I'll see if Loren will take the babysitter home."

She didn't say a word, but I knew what she was thinking.

"I don't ask for much. But it looks like we could get away from the kids just one night a year to enjoy ourselves without you having to go out and doctor on somebody's sick stock," was exactly what she was saying to herself.

As I followed Carney Sam out to his place, I thought about the many times that Jan and I had missed parties, school functions, choir practices and similar activities because of conflicting animal emergencies. I was thankful that she understood the nature of our profession, even though she often was disappointed. Since I was the only vet in the county and these people were my clients, "inconvenient" emergencies were just part of my job, even though I didn't always like it.

There was a dim light in the old barn, so I knew that Werner Fred was sitting up, nervously waiting on Carney Sam to return with the doctor.

"Izzat 'chu, Daddy?" a voice asked from the corner stall. "Ah'm down here wi' Dixie."

Dixie was lying quietly on the stall floor, covered with sweat and lather. Her abdomen was bloated badly, and there were abrasions and big bruises on the poor beast's head where she had been flopping around in pain.

"Daddy, she finally got easy 'bout an hour ago, but now she won't git up," Werner Fred allowed.

When I examined the old mare, I found that her gums were kind of murky blue, her ears were ice cold, her pulse was thready and 120 per minute and there were no intestinal sounds. She was in deep shock, probably from a ruptured stomach or intestine. It was all over for her, but how was I going to break the news to her master that she surely would be dead by morning? I looked at Carney Sam and shook my head.

Somewhere in my training I must have been absent the day they taught us how to diplomatically deliver the news to animal owners that their dog or horse is not going to survive. It is a dreaded and difficult task for me, especially if that owner is not mentally prepared for the bad news.

Werner Fred didn't realize that the mare was quiet now because her stomach had ruptured, and she finally was easy because of severe and terminal shock. I suspect that Carney Sam knew that, but he was going to make me tell his son all about it.

"Carney Sam," I asked, "would you go get me a bucket of warm water?"

I knew that he would have to heat the water in a kettle on the wood stove and then dilute the hot with cold, hand-drawn well water. Actually, I just wanted to get him out of the stall so I could tell the bad news to Werner Fred.

Good old mare . . .

"She's sure been a good old mare, hasn't she? How old is she?" I asked.

" 'Bout 20, Doc," he said without hesitation. "Ah ride her nearly ever' afternoon when Ah git home from school."

"Werner Fred," I started, "I'm afraid what I've got to

tell you is going to be bad. I'm afraid Dixie is not going to make it. She's just too sick."

The young man was tough as nails, but, when he looked up at me, there were big tears in his eyes. He was trying hard to hold them back in front of me, but his grief was just too much.

"The right thing for us to do now is to give her a shot that will just put her to sleep; then we'll know that she won't suffer any more," I said very slowly, but firmly.

He was sobbing now, as he slowly rubbed Dixie's cold and clammy neck.

"Whatever you think's best, Doc," he sobbed, "but maybe Ah betta' go ask Daddy."

"I'll go talk to him, since I need to go back to the truck anyway," I said; it was an excuse for me to leave the two together.

When I stepped up on the back porch, there sat Carney Sam in an old straight-back, cane-bottomed chair, staring into the darkness. The tough old buzzard was crying, too!

"Doc, that's why I wanted you to come out heah," he said, his voice quavering. "I just couldn't tell the boy that his hoss was gonna die. You're a heap better'n me at tellin' folks real nice like that bad things are gonna happen. Werner Fred'll believe anything you say."

"Well, I've got to put her down, Carney, if that's okay with you."

"You do what's got to be done, Doc," he said sadly. "I'll git some folks to he'p me move 'er tomorrow morning."

It always is disappointing to put an extremely ill animal to sleep. However, considering the alternative, it often is the best and most humane solution.

Werner Fred insisted on helping me inject the overdose of euthanasia solution into Dixie. Within a couple of minutes, she had quietly quit breathing, and her heart had stopped. The young man broke the silence.

"Doc, thanks for what you done," he said quietly. "I know she's a heap better off now, but Ah'll jes' always be thankful that she lived as long as she did on this farm."

Veterinarians encounter a lot of cases like Dixie. Just like leaving a midnight dance to make a call, we know what we have to do in hopeless cases, even though we don't always like doing it.

32

"Daddy, there's a cow on the patio!"

My family and I are very fortunate to be able to reside in the country. Actually, we live in the sticks! But we enjoy the space, the unpolluted air, the wildlife and the good neighbors.

Many of our neighbors are also part-time farmers. They have some cattle, pigs, sheep, a horse or two, and the usual dogs and cats, so they often call at night or on weekends for a little free advice on animal health matters. In fact, they often call in the middle of the night about problems not remotely related to health matters. So, in the interest of community harmony and neighborly goodwill, I try to help out, like a good neighbor should.

One night several months ago, I was happily dreaming about the new red and black four-wheel drive pickup truck that I want, when the phone rang. The brightly glowing digital clock projected on the ceiling that it was 11:34 p.m.

"Doc, have you got one of them tranquilizer shootin' guns on you?" a familiar neighborhood voice shouted excitedly.

I recognized the voice as that of Paul Dawson. He was a successful building supply store owner and is semiretired. Recently he had decided to raise purebred Simmental cattle, and I had been to his place several times, both officially and unofficially, to help him with various matters.

"Paul, we don't even own one," I declared. "What's wrong?"

"That new yearling bull that I bought the other day has torn down the line fence and is scaring folks to death over in Waverly Woods subdivision," he allowed.

Just a few days earlier I had Bang's and TB tested and vaccinated "Rebel." He was a handsome bull, tipping the scales at about 800 pounds. He was not mean; yet his de-

123

portment could stand considerable improvement.

The pasture where Rebel resided was right next to the ritzy subdivision. Mercedes-driving, perpetually grinning Amway salesmen, northern-university-trained English professors and well-heeled plumbing contractors are the types who eat, sleep and cut grass there. There also are some veterinary school professors who live there, but they are relegated to the back side of the property, across the dirt road from the turkey farm.

Some of the residents there seem to think that milk originates at the store and that T-bone steaks and pork chops appear magically from thin air into the supermarket coolers. Their knowledge of the food supply chain is limited, but they do know that they definitely do not like to sniff pasture or barnyard aromas while barbecuing hamburgers or rolled rump roasts on their expensive grills. The last thing they want to see or hear is a bull on their immaculately cut grass.

As I turned into the subdivision entrance, I was amazed at the enormity of the gathering and its accompanying commotion. There were several police cars cross-ways in the road, all with the blue lights flashing and some with spotlights penetrating the pine trees. Two-way radios were blaring out their staticky late-night messages.

Several pickup trucks with whips, hot shots, and coiled up cheap grass ropes hanging from gun racks were slowly cruising down the street, while the cowboy-hatted and brew-slurping occupants peered anxiously out all the open windows for signs of the culprit bull. I could see several other cowboys sauntering through yards, trying to get the kinks out of their ropes and occasionally sending healthy streams of coffee-colored tobacco juice exiting between chapped lips.

The term "cowboy" in this situation is used quite loosely to describe the individuals involved in the chase. It is true that the aforementioned cowboys drive pickup trucks rigged up with gun racks. But they either found the wide-brimmed straw hats they were wearing or picked them up last winter during a blue light special at the K-Mart. Their boots were mostly Nashville culls, had high heels and steel toes.

"Yonder he is!" one beery-breathed rope toter shouted,

as Rebel suddenly appeared and refreshed himself at a bird bath. He took one look, sniffed the situation, and immediately streaked for the woods with approximately 10 whooping and hollering cowboys in hot pursuit.

The events that followed were closely akin to a Keystone Kops episode. Within seconds, two of the cowboys were casualties from an encounter with an invisible clothesline. Holding their throats, gagging, and staggering, they hastily retreated to the safety of the pickup. Four others were rudely and stickily greeted by a row of full-grown cactus plants at the property line, and they too quickly dispatched themselves to the safety of the observation area. By now, the number of vehicles and rubberneckers on the side streets had doubled and the county mounty policemen grudgingly exited their patrol cars and commenced directing traffic as if they had suddenly been plucked up and placed down in New York City.

With nylon lariat in one hand and flashlight in the other, I joined in the chase. As I drew closer to the bull interceptor patrol, I decided to offer some advice.

"Shut up that yellin' and quit runnin' or we'll never catch him!" I offered, authoritatively.

"Who said dat?" a drunken voice echoed through the darkness, just as two other strange, yet tell-tale noises competed for attention.

"Ka-slosh! Ka-slosh!"

In the darkness, two more casualties were claimed by a new unfenced swimming pool. The victims were sloshing around frantically in the water, trying desperately to swim towards land that they could barely see. Now, lights were being flipped on in the pool owners' bedroom, followed momentarily by patio and underwater lights. The sloshing-around cowboys looked like drowning rats, barely keeping their moustached faces above water as their heavy cowboy boots kept pulling them back under. The pajama-clad owner was angrily standing in the doorway, with hands on hips and mouth agape, wondering who had the audacity to dive, fully clothed, into his prized pool without permission.

Only three left . . .

When he whirled and charged back into the house mumbling something about a shotgun, I sprinted in the opposite direction in an effort to avoid personal bloodshed. As far as I know, the swimmers saved themselves.

At this point, there were only three participants remaining in the chase — Rebel, me, and a guy named Buck.

"Over here, Doc," I heard Buck call softly, "he's up on the patio."

Sure enough, I could see old Reb's shadow on the patio of the biggest, fanciest house in the entire subdivision. I could hear nibbling and chewing noises as he snapped off and snacked on ferns in hanging baskets, weeping figs in fine pots and other prized plants. I could also hear the unmistakeable "splat, splat, splat" sounds of a bull relieving himself on the immaculate concrete floor of the patio. Bulls have absolutely no "couth" when it comes to their toilet manners.

"Daddy, there's a big old cow on the patio!" shrieked a teenager, as she jerked open a sliding glass door. Rebel took a quick peek at her, then kicked and stomped on most of the plants that he hadn't sampled, before making a quick getaway across the road and into the soybean field.

Now we had him! The triangular field funneled downhill into a small pasture with a wide gate. If someone could just go around and open the gate, then Rebel probably would just trot into the security of the well-fenced pasture. I could see Paul's truck heading lickety-split for the gate.

The only problem now was getting the cooperation of the pasture owner, one Dr. Stanley Vezey, a wealthy and brilliant, but cranky veterinarian who spends most of his time doctoring on chickens and partridges. I knew him quite well, since we shared an office together for several years. Stan goes to bed early and does not like being disturbed for any reason once the lights go out. He has been known to occasionally exhibit the business end of a shotgun to uninvited, nocturnal intruders. So when I saw Stan's yard light up like a prison compound, I was afraid we were in a passel of trouble. Sure enough, I heard the intimidating "chang, chang" sound of a shell entering the chamber of an old Remington pump.

"Who is it?" Stanley yelled from his doorstep. "What are ya'll doin' down there in my pasture? Speak up or I'll shoot!"

"Nothin', Mister," I replied in a high-pitched and

squeaky, disguised voice. "Our little, you know, bully, just hopped right out of our, you know, truck, and we've just shooed him into your, you know, nice pasture. Will it be OK if we leave him there, you know, overnight?"

"Well, yeah, I reckon," replied Stan curtly. "I don't guess he'll eat much in that length of time."

"Thanks, Mister, you're a real, you know, sweetie pie!" I gushed, in the same high voice.

Stan quickly fled back into the protection of his southern mansion and extinguished all lights. For once he was at a loss for words.

Rebel was caught up the next day with the aid of several "real" cowboys. He has grown considerably since that event, but has not broken down anymore fences since the patio incident.

I saw Stanley at a veterinary meeting a few weeks ago. During the attitude adjustment hour, I enjoyed a conversation with him. We talked about training bird dogs, the price of broilers and how to load your own shotgun shells, among other things. When we were ready to part company, I had to see what his reaction was to a certain statement.

"Mister, you're a real, you know, sweetie pie!" I said in a high pitched, squeaky, disguised voice. I then plunged into the mass of conversing vets. Looking back from the safety of the snack table, I could see Stan scratching his red head, with brow furrowing, and a strange gaze on his face. Suddenly his mouth dropped open and he quickly pointed his finger at me.

"McCormack, I'll get you for this, you redneck clod!," he declared.

I could not control my laughter. Rebel and I had put one over on Stan Vezey. Not many folks have ever done that!

33

"Don't you get my new car muddy!"

IT HAD been such a beautiful, shiny new car just an hour or so before. Now it was completely covered with brown mud and clay. There was no sign of the once beautiful whitewalls or the mirror-like expensive hubcaps.

The windshield was so dirty that there was only a cleaned-off spot about the size of a horse's foot for the driver's vision. Never has a vehicle been so muddy.

"Boy, Momma's gonna be real mad when she sees her new car," allowed Tom, the 7-year-old, as we slowly walked round and round the vehicle.

"Yeah, real mad!" echoed Lisa as she followed. She was 5. We all shook our heads in dismay and disbelief.

It was a fire engine red, four-door Buick, and it was Jan's pride and joy. We had decided to trade in the old Chevy wagon for a nicer vehicle that fall. The practice was prospering, and our clients were paying their bills exceptionally well. Even I. C. Goodmilk, the slowest payer of all, had come in and completely paid up his account.

"I don't wanna see no more bills from you for a long time, Doc," he chirped, " 'specially them with nasty notes scribbled on 'em!"

"What a blessin'," I said, staring at the check in disbelief. "You rob a bank, I. C., or did your wife go to work at the girdle factory?"

Meantime, my faithful practice truck had developed transmission trouble, and my mechanic buddy had towed it into his shop for a quick weekend repair. Reluctantly, Jan finally had agreed to allow me to use her car for my farm calls.

"Don't you dare get it dirty," she warned, "and don't be going up any of those muddy roads that are waiting to be blacktopped!"

Saturday had been fine. The calls I made were all on paved roads and I had no need to drive through pastures, harvested cornfields or cleared off new ground. Sunday morning had also been quiet. I had made only two calls before preaching and even had time to hose the auto off before going to church.

The phone was ringing when we had walked into the house at noon. It was Mr. Hugo Houston with a sick cow. She had broken into the corn crib and made herself sick by gluttonizing on ear corn.

"The road's kinda slick, Doc, so be careful," he warned.

"Is it muddy?" I asked cautiously.

"Aw, naw, that clay base is good and solid, but we did have a shower last night. We were in hopes that the county would get it paved before winter. You know what a time I've had with the commissioner about this road."

When we get ready to pave a road in the South, we build up a nice hard base with red clay, then wait for it to rain. A downpour of several inches can be depended upon in the 24-hour period just prior to the paving date. After the rain, the road's surface resembles tomato soup into which someone has scooped vast quantities of brown goo and numerous large undissolvable clods. Small pickup trucks and cars have been known to disappear into some of the large holes that appear because the surface was not packed down hard enough at that spot. Unknown to me, this was the condition of the road to Mr. Houston's place.

Tom and Lisa both begged to ride with me on the call, but Jan elected to stay home with Paul, who was only beginning to walk. They raced for the car to secure a prized front window seat.

"Y'all be careful with my car," Jan reminded as we motored out the driveway. "No mud on the floormats. Lisa, don't stand on the seats. Watch out for flying rocks, and . . ." her voice trailed off as we quickly motored out of her range.

The road really wasn't that bad. There were scattered mud holes, which we couldn't avoid, but the vehicle was only moderately caked with mud when we arrived at the farm. But, as we tromped into the barn where the cow was stalled, I noticed a dark cloud hurrying in from the southwest. It had "deluge" written all over it.

"Daddy, it's thundering!" announced Lisa a few minutes later, as I passed the stomach tube down the cow's gullet.

"Daddy, look at that rain coming!" bulletined Tom a few minutes later. I began to hurry.

Sure enough, I could hear the roar of the cloudburst, and it seemed to be following every curve and depression of the road at a very fast pace. One minute later, the mighty deluge detonated on the tin roof of the old barn. Tom and Lisa both slowly inched up to my side and secured themselves to a leg as the deafening noise of millions of plummeting raindrops tap danced just a few feet above our heads. I could see Mr. Houston's lips moving as he tried to converse, but I could hear no sound other than that of the hubbub above.

Finally it was over, and we discussed the aftercare of the cow as we emerged from the shady protection of the barn. The ground had turned to pure mud from the inch of precipitation. I knew that some of that mud would be deposited on the black floor mats and carpet of the car.

The road reminded me of a war zone route. Ditches were overflowing with muddy water everywhere, and there were limbs and sticks strowed randomly over the road surface. I would not have been worried if I had been in my faithful truck, since it was famous for negotiating almost impossible roads. Nevertheless, I gunned the accelerator and spun out into what I thought was the middle of the road.

"Hang on, partners!" I bravely exclaimed to Tom and Lisa. They were both quietly sitting on the edge of the front seat, wide-eyed, and gripping the dash with white-knuckled tenacity.

In order to prevent getting stuck, I was traveling at a higher rate of speed than what most people would have thought appropriate. As the car slipped and splashed rapidly homeward, it would occasionally try to swap ends, which necessitated constant combat with the steering wheel. The rear end would slide crazily to the right, so I would viciously turn and whirl the steering wheel to the right. Then, because of overcompensation, the rear end would veer off to the left, getting out of the ruts where it needed to track. At the same time, the front wheels were bursting through wading pool-sized water holes, which sent the rust colored water geysering skyward and then splashing back down on the total vehicle. Since I could not stop and clean off the windshield, I found that poking my head out the window was necessary in order to see anything. Luckily, we met no other vehicle. When we arrived at the main road, I stopped just long enough to smear out a semiclean spot on the windshield. Finally we arrived at the clinic.

As we continued walking around the filthy car, we formulated a plan. Since we were parked at the side of the clinic, we would just clean it up right there, then take it home. Perhaps Jan would never know!

"Tom, you go get the hose from the kennels, and turn on the water full blast. Lisa, you get the floor mats out, and then go get the Ajax cleanser from under the bathroom sink. Somebody get a boot brush!" I ordered. Now it was becoming a game, to see if we could get away with it.

For 45 minutes we hosed, splashed, scrubbed, scraped, swept and wiped. The soil conservation man would have been appalled if he had seen the soil that we washed out from under the car as well as from on top. Next, we took towels from the clinic and wiped it dry.

Finally, we stood back by the hedges guarding the road and marveled at our handiwork.

"I never thought it would come clean!" I said happily.

"Me neither," agreed Tom.

"Me neither," echoed Lisa.

"Tell you what, boys and girls," I said in a whisper, as I knelt down and put my arms around them. "It probably would be better if we didn't mention this to Momma. This will be sort of our special little secret, O.K.?" We all clasped our hands together and made "Shhh" noises with our fingers to our mouths.

Jan was sitting on the front porch crocheting one of her beautiful and famous afghans when we drove up into the carport. Paul was asleep in his playpen at her side. She was carside within seconds with hands on hips and a crocheting needle crossways in her mouth.

"I'll never, ever loan my car out again!" she exploded. "You can't have anything around here without somebody messing it up!"

"Wait a minute, dear! What's wrong?" I asked, as the kids and I stared at each other.

"Just look," she said, "there's a spot of mud on that right rear hubcap. And look, there's another spot on the radio antenna. What's that small kudzu leaf doing sticking in there beside the headlight?"

"Just calm down, dear!" I allowed. "Tell you what. The kids and I will take the hose and clean off those little spots, and it will look as good as new."

Five minutes later, after making a great show of washing and drying, I asked for her opinion.

"It does look so pretty, just like when it left here a couple of hours ago. I just knew that you were going to take it off on some muddy road and get filth all over it. I apologize."

"Oh, that's all right, Jan," I said, as I winked at the kids and they grinned with hands over their mouths. "We forgive you for doubting us."

She'll never know the truth. Unless she reads this, of course.

34

A freaky Saturday night

IT WAS a pleasant Saturday evening in October. The oaks
and hickories were changing their colors, and the cool west
Alabama air smelled of cotton picking time and football
games. I had looked forward to that particular day for several weeks since I had heard that Auburn was going to play
Tennessee on TV that night. I was hoping that just once, I
could sit quietly with my family and enjoy watching a good
football game without interruption. Kind of like a normal
family might do.

On my way back into the clinic from a call south of town,
my wife called me on the two-way.

"Mr. Clinch is on the phone," she said in her always
pleasant telephone and radio voice, "and one of his best
cows has been in labor all day. He wants you to come see
about her."

Mr. Clinch was one of my best clients. He had 300 sows,
200 Santa Gertrudis cows, a dozen or more coon dogs and a
fine lake full of bream and bass. The only problem was
that his farm was 45 hard-driving, dusty road miles away
in the neighboring county to the north.

Well, there went the game. It was 6 o'clock, and by the
time I drove 90 miles round trip and got the calf delivered,
it would be halftime, at the earliest. Perhaps I could get
home in time to see the second half.

"O.K., Chief," I said. "How about telling him to hang up
the phone and watch for a cloud of dust. I'm on my way!"

The trip to the Clinch farm wasn't too bad since it was
too early for the stateline drunks to head home for the
evening and too late for the road-hogging pulpwood truck
traffic.

Upon arriving at the farm, Mr. Clinch was nowhere to be
seen. Instead, one of his part-time helpers, B. J. Roach,

was sitting on the corral fence. The cow was penned up, which was an unexpected delight, but I would be doing everything by myself since B. J. was worthless when it came to helping treat sick stock.

"Mr. Clinch, he said to tell you that the cow is in the pen, Mr. Doc," B. J. said, loudly.

"Where's he, B. J.?" I asked.

"I think he's over there with that country club crowd watching 'at football game on the television, Mr. Doc," he said.

"Now isn't that something!" I thought to myself. "Here I am bustin' a gut trying to help this cattleman, while he's over at the fancy country club having a ball and watching the big game on color TV, no doubt!"

"Go get me a bucket of water, please, B. J." I requested. Maybe I could get in the catch pen and have the calf delivered before he got back with the water.

The patient was an older cow, which was surprising, since most O.B. cases are first-calf heifers. She did not offer to get up when I climbed over the fence into the corral, placed the lariat over her head and made it into a temporary halter. As I was getting the rope fixed over her nose just right, she stood up but still didn't offer to fight, like most Brahma-blooded, O.B. cases seemed to always do on Saturday night.

When I looked at the cow from the rear, I saw two fetal feet protruding, with their soles pointing down.

"Aha," I thought happily, "betcha it's just a retained head. Me and my trusty calf saver snare will have this thing out of here in minutes few!"

After washing up the appropriate areas, I made my examination. Sure enough, the fetal head was crooked around and lying along the right side of the fetal body. My long arms were sure going to come in handy on this case.

"B. J., would you go to the truck and turn on the switch so we can listen to the ball game while we work?" I requested.

As I introduced the snare to retrieve the head, Auburn kicked off. Getting the thing manipulated into the right spot and over the poll wasn't quite as easy as I had anticipated. The object of my immediate search was just barely out of my reach, and just when I thought I had the head in my grasp, the snare would slip off. About the same time, Auburn would fumble or get penalized for interference, or the quarterback would throw an interception. That would add to my frustration and also cause me to become more depressed and tired.

The cow had decided that standing up was too difficult, so she laid back down, so she would be more comfy, I suppose. Now I was lying down on my side and on my stomach in the dirty lot, straining and pushing, trying to accomplish my objective. I had replaced the snare with a 60-inch O.B. chain, now, and looped it around the lower jaw.

"Pull on this chain with that handle, B. J." I said, "and let's see if we can get this head straightened out."

He jerked the thing too hard, though, and went sprawling backward when the loop didn't hold. He did extract two teeth with his mighty pull.

When I again tried to get the chain looped on the head, I discovered that the lower jaw contained all its teeth! After all that struggling, I realized then that I was dealing with a two-headed fetus. No wonder I couldn't get it to budge! I'd have to do a cesarian now to get this monster delivered.

The football game on the radio was having problems, too. According to the announcer, it was total war, with many casualties being suffered by both sides. As I prepared the cow for surgery, they took one player off the field on a stretcher, and another wobbled off in a confused mental state. The announcer kept going on about what a great game it was. Why couldn't I have been in my home enjoying it like everyone else in the country?

As the surgery progressed, the radio became more and more staticky, and the broadcaster's voice finally faded completely away. The last thing I heard him say was something about a minor misunderstanding on the field turning into a major fracas involving both benches, coaches and some slightly toxic fans.

Finally, I made the incision into the calf bed and gazed upon the cause of all the poor cow's trouble. B. J. was suddenly at cowside, gasping and pointing at the freakish fetus, after about a 20-minute absence due to nausea and light headedness.

"Whoo-wee!" marveled the pale-faced B. J., "I ain't never seen nothin' like 'at. Wait'll I tell everybody at the feed store Monday about this two-headed monster!"

Extracting the fetus and closing the incisions was un-eventful. B. J. was rattling on and on about the happening and how "we" had done this or that, and how he figured all along that the cause of the problem was a freak. All of a sudden he was an expert. I was suturing as fast as I could, wanting to get away from his incessant chattering and get in my truck so I could find out about the ball game.

On the way home, I could find no radio stations that were reporting football scores. But when I arrived home, my wife had a report for me.

"Oh, so many of the nice young men were badly hurt, and there was a terrible brawl that involved both squads. It was quite a game!"

"Well, who won, who won?" I asked quickly.

"Oh, I don't know about that," she said. "I changed channels during that horrible fight and started watching Lawrence Welk."

A quick phone call to one of my buddies gave me the dope on the game. I could have waited until the following week and read about the two Saturday evening events in the weekly paper. There on page two were two pictures. One was a photograph of the big football game fight, and the other was of a grinning B. J. holding up the two-headed calf. The article stated that Mr. B. J. Roach, head herds-man at Clinch Farm, had delivered the freak calf. He had also told the newspaper that the event was a rarity in his vast experience, and that it occurred about once in every 10,000 births.

Not one word about the sore-muscled veterinarian who had wallowed around on the ground, groping, groaning, pushing and straining for an hour. No mention was made of the fine surgery done by the doctor, nor the fact that the cow had survived and was doing well. *Nothing* was said about the vet spending his entire Saturday evening doing all that hard work and missing the big game on TV. It didn't state that the owner was not even present for the birthing or that he was over at the country club.

That was O.K. with me, though, since I took all of it into consideration when I made out the bill!

35

Remembering Old Ada

I CLEARLY can remember sitting proudly on her back when I was 4 years old. She would have been about 20 years old at the time, and I can recall that she was all decked out in her working gear — collar, a new back band, trace chains, and so on. I had taken a small keg of cool spring water to my dad, who was working with the old mule in the scorching hot cotton field, and my reward was a short ride atop "Old Ada."

As mules go, Ada wasn't much to look at. She was black with a light gray muzzle and had the long ears so characteristic of mules. Her lower lip always dangled and she drooled a lot. I suspect that she had suffered some kind of nerve paralysis to her tongue or other mouth parts that caused the abnormality. She had those real sad eyes that gave the appearance she was always grieving over something.

Ada and my dad had started farming together in the 1920's. As far as I know, tractors were practically nonexistent back then in the small cotton fields of southern middle Tennessee. All the field work was done by mules, or in some cases, horses. Land was turned, corn and cotton planted, cultivated and harvested, all with mules. Hay was cut, hauled to the barn and lifted into the loft with a large single or double hay fork with those equine beasts of burden. We hauled river gravel to spread on the roads, hauled cotton to the gin, and some people even went to town and church in a wagon pulled by a team of mules.

I assume that all young farm boys want to be like their dads and want to do what their dads do. I know that I did. I admired the way that he could hand milk a short-teated cow so quickly, could gear up a team of mules and tie those hamestrings so tight and pretty, and the way that he could plant a corn or cotton row so arrow straight.

But the thing that was the greatest to me was the way he could handle those mules and get them to do what he wanted done. It looked so easy! With a "haw" here and "yea" there (we said "yea" instead of "gee"), an occasional mouth cluck and a light tap with the lines every now and then, he could have those mules tiptoeing through cotton rows like Fred Astaire, never stomping on a stalk.

So, I just couldn't wait until I was old enough to "bust out" cotton middles with Old Ada. After that, I was just sure I quickly would be elevated to handling a team of mules all by myself.

Long before I was ready to plow by myself, Dad would let me hold the plow handles and plow lines, while he walked to the side or just behind me. I realized then that it wasn't going to be as easy as I had first thought.

That's where Ada took over. She had a knack for training young boys and men to the plow. The first time she and I worked together alone, I yeaed and hawed, yelled, slapped her with the reins, but all she did was to do as she pleased, and look around at me in disgust when we got to the end of each row. That was when I found out that mules weren't anywhere near as dumb as everyone thought. How else could Old Ada walk through the middle of a cotton row, around rocks and stumps, yet never damage a single cotton plant?

One time we were going down through a cotton middle with a bull tongue plow when she slowed down and stopped for some reason. I angrily slapped the reins and said, "Come up!" She did as she was told and about two seconds later a below-ground stump caught the plow point and stopped us on a dime. Those of you who have never been jabbed in the lower abdomen by a plow handle have been very fortunate. While I was doubled up in what I thought was terminal pain, Ada just looked around and snickered. I know that she was laughing because her eyes were half closed and her lips were quivering. From that day on, I stopped when she stopped!

Ada was a loner. She did not like other equines, cows, calves or barn cats. She and I got along real well, since I was the one who usually fed her a few ears of corn and a flake or two of hay every day. The low point in her life

138

came the day Dad bought a team of gray mares named Nelle and Belle. These horses would have easily qualified for the Olympic stubborn team. And Old Ada hated them, probably because they harrassed her so much. Nelle's first stall was right next to Ada's, but Dad had to move Nelle across the barn hall, since there was so much commotion. Nelle tried to bite Ada through the stall partition, tried to kick the wall down to get to her, and continually harrassed her next door roommate in every manner possible.

When a cat would make the mistake of trying to pay Ada a visit, Nelle would try to kick, stomp, or otherwise eliminate the unwanted visitor. More than once she bit a Jersey calf on the top of her neck when the young bovine came too close.

As tractors and other mechanical implements gradually took over more and more of the farm chores, Ada was called upon to do less and less work. Plowing the garden was probably the biggest job she carried out in her old age. Eventually, she did nothing other than loll around in the large hilly and rocky lot behind the barn. When I would get off the school bus and walk down the hill past the lot toward the house, Ada would meet me at the barn and escort me down the road as far as she could. When someone asked Dad why he didn't just get rid of the old mule, he would quickly reject the notion.

"No siree!" he'd explain. "She'll live out her life right here on this place. She's done too much for my family for me to sell her off like a worn-out piece of equipment."

The last time I saw her she was standing under one of the old pignut hickory trees in her private lot. I was off to college, and I really never wanted to walk behind mules again, especially if they were pulling a Barton harrow or hillside plow. There were later times, though, when I would be slaving over a term paper or studying for an organic chemistry test that I would have gladly traded places with a plow hand.

Not long after I had left home, one of my mother's letters related the bad news.

"We found Old Ada dead in her stall yesterday morning," she wrote. "She got down Sunday and couldn't get up. Daddy and Shannon buried her over on the back side of Ardmore hill. I guess it was just old age."

139

I remember going to my fourth floor dormitory room and just staring out of the window, looking out across the Tennessee River. I realized how much Ada had meant to our family and how hard she had slaved in the fields in order that we could have a living. I probably would not have even gone to college if it hadn't been for her. Even full-grown men can shed unashamed tears over an old mule.

Now years later, as I look back, I know that Ada taught me several valuable lessons. The first was that if you need a job done right, get a work horse, not a show horse. Also from her I learned consistency. She was always the same, every day, regardless of the situation. She was dependable, persistent, and always did a little more than her share. Aren't those all attributes that we all strive to attain? Isn't it odd that we can learn these lessons from an old mule?

36

A bad kind of runt pig

FRED was born over a year ago, a runt. He's still a runt and always will be a runt unless some brilliant high-tech university scientist quickly comes up with some dramatic cure for that dreaded malady, porcine runtism.

Fred's parents cannot be faulted. His father, a strapping 500-pounder of Duroc ancestry, is the picture of health. Bulldog, his spotted Poland-China-type mother, also has a curly tail, pink gums and clear eyes. His 11 healthy sibling littermates have long since been sliced or pattied and set before some chop-licking stranger at Morrison's or the Hilton or the Waffle House.

Neither can the management on Fred's farm be criticized. He has had the finest soybean meal and corn available placed before him twice a day in clean receptacles. His drinking water is clean and has been tested for purity and evil bacteria by the county health department. To his credit, he has done more than his share by consuming said victuals with hearty zeal and then grunting for more.

When he was 4 weeks old, Fred suffered physical trauma, as well as emotional defacement. His mother, in a moment of rage, not only tossed him from the nest with her smelly snout, but also stomped on him with one of her large cloven hooves. The wiry little porker probably avoided passing through the pearly gates by playing dead in the deep pine straw for several hours.

When his owner found him, Fred's outer claw on his left front foot was smashed and bleeding badly. Emergency first aid was attempted by the owner while her husband streaked for the phone to summon the veterinarian.

"Doc, Fred's been hurt real bad," he yelled. "Old Bulldog just stomped the little feller nearly to death! I need ya!"

Not long after the phone call, I was at Fred's side. His toe was hanging by a small strand of skin, and it was obvious that a quick snip with the scissors and a tight wrap was in order.

"This won't take but a second," I announced, reaching for an instrument.

Can't do a transplant . . .

"Wait, don't cut!" screamed Fred's landlord. "Can't you go to the slaughter house, get another toe and graft it on?"

I was stricken with deadly silence for a few moments as I pondered the unusual request. All I could do was blink my eyes and try to figure out how I was going to get this animal lover to listen to reason.

"Ma'am," I began, "I just don't have the technical know-how to perform transplant surgery, and I don't believe we can get a hold of anybody who will do it on this pig. Besides, the cost will make the procedure prohibitive."

"I don't care what it costs, dadgummit!" she retorted. "It just doesn't seem right to make my little Freddie go through the rest of his natural life with only one toe on that side!"

Have mercy! What could I say? Where was I the day of the lecture on how to talk to people who make unrealistic requests?

"Yes'm, I understand," I answered, "but this little piggy will be able to live a good life without that toe. He'll still hunt for acorns and root around in the dirt just like a normal hog, after a short period of convalescence, of course."

"What's this period of convalescence?" she asked.

"Well, you'll need to keep him up here at the barn in a private stall and give him extra attention. You'll need to change the bandage on this foot every few days.

"Oh, I won't mind that," she replied. "You can depend on me to take care of my pigs. I will expect you to check in on him, though, when you are making your daily rounds."

The minor surgery was completed in short order, the foot bandaged nicely and an injection of penicillin given. Fred squealed, wiggled and squirmed like a normal pig but showed no sign of violent behavior. Little did we know that this would quickly change.

When I returned several days later, Fred looked fine as he peered suspiciously at me through the cracks in the stall door. He would greedily take a couple of slurps of his gruel, then pause briefly in his chewing and stare at me intently.

When I opened the door and stepped into the stall, the rascal charged at me like a wild Mexican bull! He actually went for my right ankle, with fangs flashing! With shock and surprise I exited the stall with dispatch.

I have been attacked by dogs, cows, bulls, parakeets, sneaky rams, sows with pigs and farmers, but never by a 10-pound pig!

"What's happenin', Doc?" asked the farm proprietress as she walked up.

"Yo' little Fred attacked me!" I announced. "Just look at these slobber marks on my coveralls!"

She looked, and then she laughed. Now I often laugh at myself and usually join in the guffawing when I make a dumb mistake. But I detest being laughed at when I've just been attacked by a vicious beast, even if the beast is no bigger than a south Georgia turnip.

"I'll catch him," she offered, "seeing as how you are scared of the little fella."

"Wonderful," I mumbled.

She immediately hopped into the stall as she made proper porcine noises with her mouth. It was obvious that she was experienced in communicating with swine.

Went for her ankle . . .

Fred had backed into the corner, trying to hide. But, when he saw the second human leg in less than five minutes invade his territory, he jumped on it with equal little-pig vigor.

"You little three legged, runty sapsucker!" she yelled as she jumped from the stall. "I oughta git me a club an' work on yo' head!"

I laughed with great gusto.

We finally caught Fred by locating a piece of plywood and trapping him in the corner of the stall. By then, the owner had really become red-faced with anger, so she was able to catch Fred easily and hold him in a wrestling-like neck and leg lock while I treated his foot.

This routine was repeated several more times when we treated his foot. Each time the conflict resulted in flared tempers on both sides, and I would be ill as a hornet the rest of that day.

Fred recovered nicely and is no longer lame. He does torment his porcine colleagues on the farm, however, evidence that his temperament has not improved.

37

Four-word sentences vets hate to hear

LIFE is like a roller coaster ride — a series of ups and downs, of highs and lows. Some days everything goes right for us veterinarians, while other days are filled with one disaster after another. It is easy to let the disaster days get a person down, especially if one is easily depressed or that bad day happens to be a Monday. Often a four-word sentence over the telephone can instigate a feeling of depression.

"She died last night." It is always depressing to lose an animal, especially when I have predicted that she will survive. Contrary to the belief of many farmers, buzzards do not fly along behind us licking their chops and with bibs tucked in. Some days, however, I do scan the skies for those pesky vultures.

I've found that livestock owners don't expect their vet always to save an animal, but they do expect us to make a strong effort and be able to consistently predict the outcome of any given case. A cow down, toxic, and dehydrated with coliform mastitis has a relatively poor chance of survival. So has a downer from malnutrition, perforated and badly bleeding abomasal ulcers, a calf with a brain abscess or advanced fatty liver disease.

On the other hand, metritis, left displaced abomasum or primary ketosis cases have a good prognosis if attended to without delay. The ability to prognosticate the outcome of cases takes experience, as well as a good "cow sense."

"You're too late, Doc." I've gone through the traffic light, nearly run down the town drunk, thrown gravel into the preacher's windshield and exceeded the speed limit by 50 miles per hour to get to the bloated or prolapsed cow. With steam billowing out from under the hood and my eyes dilated widely, these four words always are a letdown.

145

I once left a pen full of unvaccinated cattle to drive 30 miles to see a "horse dyin' with the colic!" When I finally skidded to a stop in front of the stable, I saw a bloated horse piled onto a front end loader.

"You're too late, Doc," sneered the owner.

"When did she expire?" I asked.

"Aw, yesterday, about bull bat time," replied the owner.

"Well, why did you call just a while ago in a panic?" I asked in a diplomatic manner.

"Well, we thought maybe you could see if the other horse was gonna die or not," he declared, matter-of-factly.

Meanwhile, back at the ranch, one cattleman and four cowboys are cooling their heels, whittling and telling lies till Doc gets back. The owner is getting more riled by the minute.

"We can't catch her." The call came in at 11:00 p.m. The Brahman crossbred heifer has been in labor all day but still has all the escape instincts of an enranged buck deer. Now I'm searching a stumpy and marshy pasture with headlights for Brahman eyes.

"Doc, when we find her, I'll just drive yo' truck and let you stand on the back bumper and you can lasso her from there," says the generous farmer.

"Wow!" I say to myself, "I can't wait!"

I did this number on several occasions, until I fell off that bumper one night while going 25 mph. If you've ever fallen off a vehicle moving at that speed, you will remember how many different parts of your anatomy, front and back, you can touch with your nose as you skid along the ground like a pine stump.

"Where were you yesterday?" I practiced veterinary medicine for several years in an area where my nearest colleague was 35 miles away. After working several years straight through, I decided to take a day off to see if the divorce threat was real. When I returned to work early the next morning, there was a note upon my door, curtly requesting my presence at a certain farm to relieve a heifer dystocia. When I arrived at the farm, I was grilled thoroughly about my whereabouts the previous day.

"We needed ye Doc, and we couldn't find ye nowhere!" they preached, with head tilted and eyes narrowed.

I've wondered about that situation and others like it. If I

was so important, why did I have to scrape and strain so much to just pay the light bill?

"Send me a bill!" The most hated and the most dreaded of all client utterances!

"I'll see you Satiddy" This one is almost as bad. I'll bet more veterinarians go broke or barely scrape by because of poor fee collections than any other reason. Paying bills is like studying algebra — once you get behind, it's sure tough to catch back up.

"You charge too much" I don't recollect ever hearing a farmer saying that vets didn't charge enough! He might have thought it, but, if so, he sure didn't say it. Practice vehicles, equipment, and drugs are high, and we've got to pay those bills to keep going.

I have had small animal owners who didn't think I charge enough, though.

"Oh, Doctor, is that all? Your charges are so reasonable," a smiling lady cooed one day after I had declawed her cats. "I would have to pay three times that in California!"

Before I could grab the bill and "refigure," the check was made out and she fled out the door with wild-eyed, clawless cats packed under both arms.

I probably have overcharged a few folks in my career, but I could count those times on one hand. The way to tell if an overcharge has been made is to watch the farmer's face as he scans the bill. If his face bleaches out, lips turn purple, nostrils flare and neck veins stand out, it is best to put the Chevrolet in DRIVE and make a hasty exit, all the time smiling broadly with teeth clenched. One day while leaving such a situation, I looked into the rear view mirror in time to see the irate farmer kick his Australian shepherd and throw rocks at the D.V.M. sign on the back of my truck.

"He jus' needs wormin'!" I've heard this statement thousands of times. It is amazing how many people think that a 50-cent worm pill will cure everything from depression to distemper. This problem is primarily one of dog and cat owners, but occasionally livestock owners will think this way, too.

"The sign ain't right." Many of my clients, in the past, always checked the almanac before calling me out for any type of surgical procedures.

"You want me to geld that hoss while I'm here?" I'd ask an owner.

"Shoot naw, Doc, the sign's in the heart!" he would exclaim with a bewildered look on his face.

He won't get any argument from me about that. I figure they'll call me when their sign is right. I just hope the sign is right for getting paid!

"Don't step there, Doc!" This usually occurs when I stop quickly by a farm just to check on a cow or something. I have on my good cowboy boots or Sunday slippers and my new grey suit. The family is waiting in the car. Suddenly, the place where I step is transformed into a bottomless pit of manure, mud and barnyard ink that stains grey pants and tan boots in an instant.

Trying to explain this accident to a mate is useless, since absolutely nothing will be able to convince her that it wasn't done on purpose. I truly suspect that boogered-up Sunday clothes have caused more nasty divorces than excessive drinking or blatant adultery.

When all is said and done though, there are a couple of nice things spoken from livestock owners that make all the negative statements worth it.

"Thanks so much, Doc," and "He's a good vet," are always good to hear, especially when they are offered sincerely.

38

Only a few good country stores are left

THIS nation would be a whole lot better off if we had fewer giant supermarkets and more small country stores.

The things you purchase might be more expensive at the smaller stores, but I think we all would have more true friends, and our mental health would be more stable. There would be fewer "big shots" around, since the regular store "sitters" would keep everybody cut down to size if they got too "uppity."

The first real country store experience that I can remember came when I was about 6 years old. I was helping my Uncle Willis custom bale hay in the vicinity of Bryson, Tenn., when noontime came. After a morning of frantically punching wires and hollering, "Block, block," I was hoarse, famished and weak as pond water. It was a welcome relief when the steady chatter of the H Farmall and the rattle of the old John Deere baler finally subsided and expired into deafening quiet.

"Let's run down to Bo Coble's store and get us a bite o' dinner," Uncle Willis declared as he trotted to the pickup. He did everything in a fast walk or a run.

Even though my ears still were ringing and roaring from the mechanical racket of the morning, they picked up his welcome announcement loud and clear.

Bo Coble's for lunch! Wow! There wasn't any item that Bo didn't have in that wonderful store! I had visited there briefly a couple of times, so I knew the general layout of the merchandise. To this day, Bo Coble's store remains the standard for my appraisal of country stores throughout the U.S.

In order to qualify as an official "country store," several basic items must be available. A drink box full of ice cold soft drinks, hoop cheese covered by its original container and sitting on the counter and the ability of the customer to purchase soda crackers in three different size packages.

Cans of sardines, Vienna sausages, a stick of bologna, pork and beans, free hot sauce and real moon pies round out the basic food items necessary for qualifying. Everything else is optional.

Atmosphere also is important. The storekeeper should be a hard-nosed but friendly sort. He also should know everybody and nearly everything, and should have a plausible answer to every question. There always should be at least one and preferably two "store sitters" who appear to be guards but are there just for customers to argue with.

The appointments should include several nail kegs, both inside around the stove and outside under the tree, for comfortable sitting whether telling lies or dining. There should be a wall-mounted, hand-operated can opener somewhere near the drink box and some empty counter space for setting drinks and edibles while on the phone.

Ah yes, the phone. It should be over on the wall where there is space for thumb tacking up professional cards. In my opinion, a country veterinarian should visit all the country stores in his area when setting up practice and display his card near the phone.

I recall the food and atmosphere at Bo Coble's store that day many years ago. I remember peeling the lid back on those Possum-brand sardines, gingerly putting a few drops of Louisiana red hot sauce on them and then consuming them on crackers. I'd still rather have them than caviar.

"Who's zat redheaded boy, Willis?" one of the sitters asked, "He any 'count?"

"Aw, that's Martha and Ed's boy. He does very well punchin' wires. I'll have 'im tyin' out when he gets a little older."

"Looks to me lack he's 'bout to white eye on ye. Ain't t'at right, boy?"

"Naw sir," I replied as I speared a sausage. "Just a little tired. But these Viennas and sardines will get me goin' again." Then I took a big swig of that 12-ounce RC Cola.

"Well, you gon' need more'n 'at, balin' weedy lespedeza hay," the sitter argued.

Store sitters always have to have the last word, and it always has to be contrary to whatever you say.

At Mrs. Ruby McCord's store, some of the world's finest sitters always are there. Carney Sam Jenkins headed the team, while Buck Tutt and Hoosier Turner were other mainstays. Carney Sam has passed on now, though, and things aren't quite the same.

"Where you headed, Doc?" Carney Sam asked me one early, cold January day. I had stopped by for some milk.

"Going up here to Cappy Lou Akins' place to doctor a sick mule," I replied. I wondered how he would be able to start an argument over a sick mule.

"They ain't no need in her payin' a high priced vet to come way out here," he started. "All 'at mule needs is some chinaberry tea and his navel turpentined."

"She wants the mule saved, not blistered to death," I said sarcastically.

"Well, that's fine if she don't mind makin' yo' truck payment fer ye this month," he said, as he and Hoosier Turner shrugged their shoulders, shook their heads and swigged on their RC's.

"Somethin' fer ye, Doctuh," Miss Ruby said, as I retrieved a quart of Borden's from the icebox and a moon pie from the bread shelf. I always waited on myself at Miss Ruby's.

"What ails Cappy Lou's mule, Doctuh?" she inquired.

"Got a touch of colic, I suspect." I bit into the pie, then washed it down with cold milk.

"If he ain't sick, he will be fo' long," I heard Hoosier mumble to Carney Sam. Both giggled and swigged as I glared at one, then the other. As I headed for the door, I decided to throw out some bait.

"Did y'all know they had to put Tootie Turner's girl in the hospital last night? You know, the one that eats all those moon pies?"

"No, no," they chirped in unison, "what's wrong with her?" They had taken the bait!

"Aw, she ate so many moon pies her stomach went into an eclipse!" I grinned, hardly able to control an explosive guffaw.

Then, before they could even close their gaping mouths, I was out the door and was bounding down the steps.

In less than five minutes, I had refreshed myself with

151

two of nature's finest products, had exchanged good na-
tured banter with friends and, to top it off, had gotten the
best of them for once. I would feel good the rest of the day!

There are only a few stores left like those owned by Bo
Coble and Mrs. Ruby McCord. Visit and enjoy them while
you can because they are a disappearing part of American
culture. They're good for what ails you!

39

"You awake, Doc?"

IT WAS in the vicinity of 3 a.m. It was very dark and the interior of my house was very quiet, except for the steady breathing of its inhabitants and the ticking of a clock.

Suddenly, the quiet was shattered by a loud ringing sound that aroused me back to a semi-conscious state. Thinking that the irritating noise was the jingling alarm clock, I tried to locate the offensive device to strangle out the noise, but knocked it off my bedside table instead.

"It's the phone, dear," my wife said. "Answer the phone!"

"Uh, oh yeah," I mumbled.

"Uh, hello," I said, speaking into one end of the thing, as the other half of the phone tumbled to the floor beside the clock.

"You awake, Doc John?" the voice asked.

"Huh? Hello?" I said, still prone.

"Doc John, you awake?" the voice then yelled.

"Oh, yeah!" I replied. "Sure. Yeah, I'm 'wake."

"Doc John, we got this yearlin' tryin' to find a calf. Can you come?"

"Uh yeah," I said with eyes still closed. "I'll be there quick as I can." Then I put the phone down somewhere, never leaving the prone position. I realized that I was hurting all over.

Several seconds elapsed before any sound was uttered.

"Who was that, Dear?" my wife asked.

I took about five seconds before it hit me. I didn't even know who the caller was! Why didn't he identify himself? Why didn't I ask who it was?

Many of my clients didn't, and still don't, identify themselves. However, I usually can figure out who is calling in a few seconds before the conversation gets too far along. Not if I'm abruptly awakened from a deep sleep, though.

The previous day had been a "bell ringer." It had been sale barn day and I had been exposed to enough work for three animal doctors. The phone had started early with a milk fever, then "Rye" Miller was injured in an automobile accident. "Rye" was one of the neighborhood dogs whose owner was one of our closest friends. I had spent an hour treating "Rye," who had a broken leg, and his owner, who had a broken heart.

Several clients came into the clinic while I was setting Rye's broken leg. Some were picking up medicine, while others were just regular drop-ins who wanted to talk football or discuss the cull cow market. I was trying to get the in-clinic dogs treated and get out of there before anything else happened.

I made two calls on the way to the auction barn 45 miles away, to deworm some horses at one place, and to calfhood vaccinate a group of wild Charolais heifers at the other.

The sale barn work that day was an experience in total chaos. My helper didn't show up for work since he was a guest in the county jail as a result of a knife fight. A substitute worker was located, but his previous work experience in a doughnut shop was not conducive to blood testing the 400 or so cows and vaccinating a pen full of feeder pigs. Mostly, he just got in my way while I madly carried out my duties.

The late night trip home was as dangerous as a hurricane. Several times I snoozed off, but would abruptly wake up when the truck ran off the road. Upon arrival at home, I collapsed into bed and was instantly asleep.

"I don't know," I replied to my wife's question about the caller's identity.

"You don't know?" she answered. "Then what are you going to do?"

"Make coffee," I mumbled as I eased my stiff and aching back out of the bed and headed for the kitchen. I reckoned that I would just wait and hope that the unknown client would call back.

While the coffee was brewing and I was thinking, the phone rang again.

"Great," I thought, "he realized that he didn't give me his name and now he is calling back."

"Doc John, I forgot to tell you that the little ol' yearlin' is in the catch pen, not in the barn."

"Wait, wait, who is this?" I pleaded. But I was too late, the phone was dead.

Now all I had to do was to figure out which one of my clients called me "Doc John," had both a catch pen and a barn, called heifers "yearlins" and had a telephone. I decided to go quickly through my accounts receivable book, read off the names and see if any of them fit the description.

Abner Abston — Everything fit except that he fed out steers only.

Biff Curtis — Dairyman that always called me "Doc John" but didn't have a catch pen.

Frank Pollock — Had a barn and a catch pen but called me "Dr. Mac."

Joe Stamps — Called heifers yearlins but didn't have a barn and refused to use a phone.

Zippy Zeigler — Bingo! He **would** be the last name in the book. But that did sound like his voice on the phone, he did have a catch pen and barn, and he sometimes called me "Doc John."

Moments later, as my white Chevy sliced through the foggy night, I was congratulating myself for the detective work I had done in figuring out who the unknown caller was.

"Just used good old-fashioned horse sense," I said to myself. "I'll bet those smart Cornell boys couldn't have figured that one out. 'Course, maybe they would have gotten his name the first time he called."

Zippy's catch pen was right beside a gravel road about a mile from his house. When I arrived at the pen, I was surprised that he wasn't there. I pulled the truck up as close as possible so the headlights would shine through the cracks.

The patient was lying down over in the corner and was in hard labor. My flashlight beam could see the evidence of her labors — a small pink nose and two tiny hooves, barely protruding from the birth canal.

With speedy enthusiasm I gathered bucket, halter, obstetrical bag and calf jack from the truck and heaved them over the corral fence. Then I was able to ease over to the

155

cow, halter her and tie her to a post before she stood up.

"This is not a yearling heifer," I thought to myself. "This is an older cow. I wonder why Zippy called her a yearlin', and I wonder why she can't have this calf? Everything looks in order."

I decided to assist with the birthing process by gently tugging on the little calf's legs with my bare hands. Almost immediately, the cow assisted with a strong contraction, and the little calf was lying at my feet, trying to get his first breath.

"That was too easy!" I thought. "Something's not right about this."

Zippy had never called with anything this simple. He usually waited until nature had been given every chance, and the patient had very little chance left for survival.

Still pondering the situation, I dipped a bucket of water from the bathtub trough, added disinfectant, scrubbed up, and examined the cow for a twin and evidence of any problems. There were none. By now, the little calf was trying to sit up and see what his new and cold environment looked like. So, I removed the halter from the cow and got out of the way.

This is a time that I especially enjoy. It is simply a miracle of nature to see a new mother cow suddenly sniff and speak tender, loving, bovine messages to her newborn baby and commence the massaging and licking action with her rough tongue. I know then that she is going to "take the calf" and that all is well.

As I stood there taking in the scene in awe and wonder, the two-way radio went off.

"Base to unit one, base to unit one," my wife's voice said, "do you read?"

"Yeah, go ahead, Jan," I replied, after I had climbed over the fence and found the microphone.

"Honey, Homer Jack Gillis wants to know where you are! He said he called an hour or so ago, and you still haven't shown up. Are you all right?"

Of course! It was Homer Jack who called, not Zippy! Now I was going to have to go clear to the opposite end of the county to his farm . . . That also meant that I had needlessly delivered a calf at Zippy's.

"Okay. I'll head on over there. I came up to Zippy Zeig-

156

ler's by mistake. Ten-four."

"John, you've just got to get home and get some rest! You are burning the candle at both ends! You know very well that you can't keep up this hectic pace very long!"

But I was busy putting my equipment back into the truck for the journey across the county.

"Do you read me, unit one?" Jan asked.

"There's a lot of static and skipping on the air tonight. I can't make out what you're saying. Ten-four."

"Never mind, I'll talk to you later. Ten-four," she said.

I tore out down the road, trying to make up for lost time.

"Why didn't I figure out that the phone caller was Homer Jack?" I wondered. He was one of my golfing buddies, so I should have recognized his voice. He wasn't in my ledger book, though, because I always sent the bill to his wealthy father-in-law.

Thirty minutes later my vehicle rocketed into Homer Jack's driveway, zoomed down the lane, and slid to a stop beside his catch pen. Homer Jack and Coo-Coo Bruce were climbing out of the corral.

"Well hello, Doc John," Coo-Coo cooed, "where you been? Did you come by way of the state line?"

"Sorry, people," I said, "since Homer Jack didn't identify himself over the phone, I didn't know where to go! Where's the heifer?"

"Aw, you're about 10 minutes too late, Doc John," said Homer Jack. "Me an' Coo-Coo already got the calf. Go on back home and git yo'sef another hour's worth of sleep. Send me a bill if I owe you anything."

"Why do these things always happen to me?" I wondered as I drove home. "I've driven all these hard miles in the dark of the early morning, only to do nothing except lose a bunch of money. I can't charge Zippy, since he didn't call me, and I was too late to help Homer Jack. I wonder if these dumb things ever happen to those Cornell vets."

The instant I realized the blue lights reflected in my rear view mirror and the siren belonged to the car to my rear, I looked down at my speedometer. It said 84 mph.

I finally stopped, then just sat there seething in disgust. I really wasn't surprised after the farcical buffoonery of the last three hours.

"Doc, you awake?" the trooper sternly asked as he arrived at my door. "You're all over this road! You been over to the state line, or what?"

Briefly, I tried to explain my problem to the patrolman. He did not seem to be sympathetic, nor was he impressed with my long working hours.

"Now Doc, you go on home and get some sleep, heah? But I don't want to see you goin' over 65 from now on! One of these nights Cap'n Simmons is gonna be patrolling this heah stretch of road an' he'll tho' you in jail in a New Yawk minute."

"I will, I will!" I promised, "I'm much obliged to you. I really am gonna slow down this time!"

"You better!" he warned as he started back to his car. Halfway there, he suddenly stopped and yelled.

"Doc, you got a flat on this left rear tire. Musta' run over a stob or somethin' up the road."

I did eventually get home, right at daybreak. Completely exhausted, I dragged myself through the back door, just as the phone rang.

"Hello," I mumbled.

"Doc, you awake . . .?"

40

Sherman's temperament was peculiar

I DON'T often see "companion" cows in my rounds as a veterinarian. However, once in a blue moon, someone will call in who has a backyard cow or steer and that animal is not existing for any economic reason. It is just there because it is the owner's pet.

One such companion animal was a bull named "Sherman." The half Charolais, half Angus giant was so named because of his mammoth dimensions. One of my students declared that he was as big as a Sherman tank. He was about the color of cold white oak ashes with an occasional splotch of brindle thrown in.

His physique was impressive. It appeared that he had been working out with weights since he was a calf and the effort had been rewarded with a "Charles Atlas" type body.

Sherman's temperament was peculiar. Around his owner, he was gentle as a kitten and would almost purr when he heard her voice. She could feed him corn out of her hand, and he would allow himself to be scratched on the head, under the belly, or in any other area. He would just stand with eyes closed and a satisfied grin on his face.

However, if a stranger would set foot into his pasture, Sherman was transformed immediately into a different bull. He would hold his head low to the ground, snort viciously, bellow loudly and shake his head wildly. His huge feet would rake dirt and send great globs of mud rocketing skyward, or would create great clouds of dust, if the weather was dry. He had been known to send blackberry pickers dashing and hollering from his pasture.

Sherman's owners were the Ramseys. They were a wealthy couple who owned the nicest restaurant in the area. Mrs. Ramsey loved animals. She had cats, dogs, horses, geese, ducks, rabbits and always was talking to sparrows as she cheerfully went about her backyard and barnyard duties.

She was a veterinarian's dream! Each animal, regardless of species, had its health monitored carefully by periodic veterinary visits and telephone consultation. I was that lucky veterinarian!

Ever since I had helped Mrs. Ramsey save some sick orphan calves and successfully treated one of her foaling mares for eclampsia, I was the only animal doctor she would allow on the place. She thought that I could cure anything!

I always dreaded working with Sherman, though. Ever since I had given him his first blackleg, IBR, BVD and anaplasmosis injections, he never had forgotten me and my needle. If he was nearby when I drove up in my white vehicle, he would immediately throw his head back and gaze at me intently while slowly and intermittently chewing on a mouthful of fescue and clover.

After a few seconds of sizing up the situation, he would start switching his tail like an angry cat and then would start marching briskly towards the farthest corner of the pasture. For that reason, Mrs. Ramsey always had him corralled whenever the schedule called for shots, deworming and fly control measures.

Usually, I would be accompanied to the farm by one or more veterinary students. When they would see Sherman angrily peering and snorting through the corral boards at the unwelcome strangers, they often would stop in their tracks as if petrified and return the stare.

"How we gon' do him?" they'd usually say, as they continued their slack-jawed stares. "He sure does look mean."

Actually, we wouldn't have "done" him if he had decided he didn't want to be "done." But Mrs. Ramsey, with feed bucket in hand, always could coax Sherman into the chute. He would smell the unmistakable aroma of cottonseed meal and crushed corn, and he would be hooked. Sometimes she would lead him into the chute with a single range cube held in her perfectly manicured hands. Sherman was a patsy for a woman's sweet talk and good food, as are most males.

160

By the time he had entered the dreaded squeeze chute, Mrs. Ramsey had slipped through the front and I had slipped a creosoted post behind him. She would reward him with the range cube or the other choice morsels and then catch his head. Trapped again!

Everybody rubbed his sides, scratched his back and cooed sweet cow talk while I quickly slapped his neck and then plunged the needles through his inch-thick hide. I really began to appreciate injectable wormers with Sherman.

It was all over before he realized what was happening. However, when his high pain threshold took priority over his voluminous appetite, his first recognizable reaction was to let out a spine-tingling and nostril-clearing nasal snort.

Find a tree . . .

"Everybody find a tree or get on the fence! Now!!" I'd order.

Students and any other spectators would burn shoe soles hunting safety. It always has amazed me how quickly a person can climb a branchless pine tree when panic strikes.

When released, Sherman always bolted from his torture chamber, trotted out into the barnyard about 20 paces and then would stop, turn around and begin his posttreatment antics. He pawed the earth, snorted, shook his head and tried to look around to see what the stinging and burning sensation was on his thick neck. This antiveterinarian demonstration would continue for some two or three minutes, and then he would trot, with big belly bouncing up and down, back into the safety of his private pasture. All this time, Mrs. Ramsey would be talking more sweet talk, but keeping her distance.

"Poor baby," she'd always say, "did Dr. John hurt my little sugar dumpling? Well, we'll just have to see about that!"

Then she would turn back towards the chute where I was standing, smile and whisper.

"Wonderful, just wonderful. You didn't hurt him a bit! He's just putting on for the students."

Looking around, I could see students up in pecan trees,

on top of the squeeze chute and one lying underneath the hay baler. Most would be holding onto something tightly and would be rigidly staring at Sherman. Their eyes would be glassy, since they had not blinked them for several minutes.

Finally, they would slowly come down from their hiding places and would start milling about, picking up the equipment we had used.

"The coffee's ready!" Mrs. Ramsey would enthusiastically declare, "and I have two fresh strawberry pies for us!"

"Ah, the benefits of working with the right kind of folks!" I'd always think to myself.

After washing up and quickly dispatching the tasty pies and coffee, we would schedule the next visit on our calendars and date books. Then we would say good-byes and head down the driveway.

One day, we were a couple of miles down the road before anyone spoke.

"Well, what do you think of that?" I asked proudly. I was hoping that someone would comment on the love Mrs. Ramsey had for Sherman, or how easily she could handle the big bull, or how expertly I had carried out the injections.

"You forgot to clean the injection site with a pledget of alcohol saturated cotton," one purse-lipped student said, "and you didn't check to see if you were in a blood vessel before you injected the vaccine. Also . . . ."

I just gripped the steering wheel tighter, bit my lower lip and counted to ten . . . .

41

Sherman, Part II

SHERMAN'S owner, Mrs. Ramsey, was very considerate of her bull's personal veterinarian. Therefore, she never called me on Sunday unless it was absolutely necessary — like if she thought he had a headache or if he looked "hollow-eyed."

One Sunday we had gone to a family reunion when she put in a call to our place. One of my colleagues, Dr. B. E. Rude, was taking my calls and emergencies while I was away. He was a good doctor and a good friend, long on veterinary knowledge and technique, but mighty short on diplomacy and tact.

As I understand it, the conversation went something like this.

"Oh, Dr. Rude, I appreciate you taking Dr. John's calls today," she said. "My fine bull, Sherman, is acting very strange, and I'm afraid that he has a ruptured appendix or something."

"Bulls don't have appendixes," he growled. "How's the old fool actin'?"

"Well, Dr. Rude," she probably said, softly, "Sherman's not a fool! He's a sweetie, and he means a great deal to me, my husband and his cow friends!"

"O.K., tell me his symptoms."

"Well, I found him lying down on the back side of the hill. He didn't want to get up, but finally did after I talked to him real sweet-like. After he got up, he would kick at his stomach, like it was hurting, then lie down and immediately get back up."

"Is that all?"

"No," she said, "he also stretches out like a horse with the kidney colic, he paws the earth and butts on the tree trunks with his head. He acts like he's going crazy with

163

pain! What do you suppose his problem is?"

"Could be lots of things."

"Well, would you be willing to take a look at him for me? I'm real worried about him. I'd just die if something were to happen to him."

"If you'll load him up and bring him over to the clinic at 4 o'clock, I'll see what I can do."

"I'll be there," she said. "I do appreciate your help and your willingness to see him."

Mrs. Ramsey always had a nice word and something nice to say about everybody, regardless of their degree of rudeness or how high up on the jerk scale they registered.

Superficial exam . . .

Dr. Rude did examine Sherman superficially between puffs of his ever-present Lucky Strike cigarette and slurps of coffee that was black as dehorning tar. But he found only that the bull was not chewing his cud. Therefore, he diagnosed "stasis of the first stomach," which was his favorite abnormal condition, and prescribed a drench of epsom salts, spiked with a few pinches of nux vomica, fenugreek and ginger.

"If he's not better by tomorrow, see if McCormack will try his luck on him," he ordered, as he slammed shut his black bag.

Sure enough, my phone was ringing at 7 a.m. the next morning. A worried Mrs. Ramsey related every aspect of the previous 24 hours and went into great detail on all Sherman's symptoms and his unsatisfactory condition.

"Dr. Rude's a wonderful man," she gushed, "but I'm just afraid that he overlooked something in Shermie." She often called him Shermie when she wanted to exhibit extra adoration.

"Oh, I do hope you can work him into your busy schedule today, this morning if possible," she pleaded.

"I'm sure we can," I said cautiously, not knowing what was on the book. "But tell me what signs he's showing now," I asked.

"Oh, he lies down most of the time, won't eat or drink, and his tummy looks pear-shaped when he stands up. Also, I'm afraid that his bowels are locked, since I have seen no evidence that they have acted."

"Uh-oh! This sounds really serious," I thought to myself. "Bet he's got some kind of G.I. tract blockage."

I dreaded the thought of having to perform abdominal surgery on Sherman. We'd surely have to put him down either on the ground or on a table. Just getting him restrained enough for proper anesthesia would be the major problem. He did not like to be held still even for a few seconds.

Down in the trailer . . .

When she arrived at the clinic, he was down in the trailer, stretched out, groaning, with his eyes walled back in his head. He looked even worse than I had anticipated.

"Shermie, please get up!" she pleaded. "Dr. John's here, sugar dumpling, and he's going to make you all better."

With that pronouncement, I walled my eyes back in my head and wondered what in the world I was going to do about this 2,000-pound downer bull with sunken eyes, bloated belly and a terrible look on his face.

After much pleading, begging, slapping and knee-gouging, Sherman arose with a nostril-clearing snort. He turned in the trailer and gave me one of those spine-tingling stares and then walked gingerly out onto the loading dock and into the Powder River chute.

"That's a good boy," cooed Mrs. Ramsey, "just put your little head in the chute and you'll be good as new in no time!" She scratched him on the head, and he closed his eyes. I walled mine again.

A quick but thorough exam revealed the problem. A long arm and rubber sleeve enabled me to palpate an intussusception deep in the right rear quadrant of the abdominal cavity. Both Sherman and I were in big trouble!

An intestinal intussusception is a complete blockage of a portion of that intestine. One portion of gut is forced down into the adjacent part, similar to the closing of a telescope. Once the telescoping occurs, the blockage is complete and final. Only rarely does the blockage "self-cure," and death is almost certain unless surgery is performed. The longer surgery is delayed, the less chance there is for survival.

Mrs. Ramsey had been following me around Sherman, wringing her hands and reassuring him that all was going to be just dandy in short order. When I listened with my stethoscope, she tiptoed quietly and motioned with her fingers to lips for Sherman also to be quiet. She looked away and cringed when I put on my long rubber sleeve and began to use it. She was so concerned! How was I going to tell her of his problem, convince her of the seriousness of it and what we had to do to correct it?

I took a deep breath and started talking in my most sincere and diplomatic manner. As I explained to the best of my knowledge and ability, she uttered nothing other than an occasional gasp and an "Oh no!" every now and then. She was trying hard not to cry, but big tears were welling up in her eyes and were beginning to streak down her perfectly-made-up cheeks. When I got to the part about the 50 percent survival rate, she started sobbing and rubbing Sherman's back briskly.

"I'm sorry, Mrs. Ramsey," I said, "but we're going to do our very best. We have good and dedicated people here to help. Perhaps he'll come through it . . ."

"Of course he'll make it," she interrupted, "of course he'll make it! I'm just so afraid that his scar will show! Can you do it where it won't show?"

I felt my eyes walling back in my head . . . again!

42

Sherman, Part III

SHERMAN was mighty sick. His blocked intestine had created a severely dehydrated, weak, toxic and halfway addled bull. Something had to be done right away.

I had a difficult time convincing Mrs. Ramsey of the seriousness of his affliction, even after a great deal of talking and drawing crude pictures of bull stomachs and other viscera on tablet paper. When she finally realized the gravity of the situation, she left Sherman in my hands and headed home for a couple of nerve pills and to lie down for a while.

My plan for Sherman was to get a bunch of folks, double halter him, get him on the surgery table, anesthetize him, make an incision into the abdominal cavity and remove the blocked portion of the intestines. While on the table, we would give him large amounts of fluids intravenously.

Our immediate problem had to do with moving Sherman from the chute to the operating table without us killing him or him killing or maiming us. It was going to be a big job.

Somehow, a wild bull always seems to draw a crowd, especially at veterinary schools. We were fortunate that day to have attracted a whole raft of students, many of whom considered themselves experts on handling any type of animal. Several others were cowboys, too, but were of the drugstore variety. They had seen cattle before, but mostly on the roadside or in picture books about Texas.

Even though Sherman was unfamiliar with rope halters, we saturated his massive head with two of them, then tied 30-foot nylon lariats onto the long end of each one. Thus, we had about 40 feet of rope to work with on each side of his head.

With approximately 10 young, lithe human bodies on each rope, we opened the chute and kindly requested Sherman to exit and to walk the 100 or so feet to the Shanks table. However, he balked and remained immobile in the chute as if his feet were set in concrete. No amount of pleading, slapping or yelling was getting the job done.

"Lemme twist his ol' tail!" tersely suggested one student, who appeared to be on leave from the football squad.

Sherman burst from the chute . . .

Suddenly, Sherman burst from the chute as if he were perilously late for "range cube time" and started loping down the alleyway with head slinging and tongue lolling. Students of every description were hanging onto their ropes with all their strength. As they grimaced and squenched their eyes shut, their tennis shoes, loafers and cowboy boots were smoking and making black marks on the concrete as they were reluctantly being dragged along. Notebooks and anatomy texts were flying into the air, and pencils and pens were being snapped in pockets like dry twigs. Horn-rimmed glasses and thermometers likewise were being trampled underfoot as the enraged beast continued his headlong rush to the surgical arena.

Then, as quickly as he had started, he slammed on his brakes and stopped dead still. The rope holders could not stop so quickly, however, and they continued on, smashing into their neighbors, the alleyway fences and the cheap aluminum gate that was hanging nearby.

As we huffed and puffed, and quickly reviewed the damage, we all wondered aloud the same thought. How can a bull that has lost 400 pounds in four days, that is 10 percent dehydrated and at death's door with a completely blocked intestine be so strong?

Before we could contemplate an answer, Sherman bolted again, catching most of the rope-holders off guard and snapping their heads back like a quickly accelerating Oldsmobile. Good news, though, this time he was heading straight for the table.

"Get the ropes tied to the table, quick!" I screamed, "and then take up the slack!"

The only problem was that the troops on the left didn't know what the word "slack" meant and they were being slung around the table viciously, while the ones on the right side were trying to take up their slack.

Finally we were able to get him up to the vertical table,

get the ropes secure and start to hydraulic the table and bull over to the horizontal.

As I wondered why things were going so well, I heard the sickening sounds of ropes being snapped. Then, in a brief chaotic eternity of approximately five seconds, the snorting bull was standing on top of the table, glaring through sunken eyes down at the 20 to 30 upward-gazing and dumbstruck students and instructors.

"This just ain't workin'," sighed one student as he dropped his rope. "I gotta go to class."

"Me, too," said another.

"You people aren't goin' anywhere 'til you help me get this bull off this table!" I asserted in a very loud, shaky voice. My temper index had risen a few notches after the events of the past half a minute.

"We'll just have to give him some Rompun, then slide him off the table onto a mat and do the surgery right here on the floor," I said as I reached for needle and syringe.

He hardly flinched as I popped him with a small dose of the sedative, but he did turn and look in my general direction. Usually, most cattle become sleepy and lie down within five minutes after the injection. Not Sherman. He required five times the regular dose before he slid off the tilted table onto the floor mat.

As several people began tying up his legs, others began IV fluids, while still others were clipping the hair off his left side. After a quick couple of skin scrubs, we injected a local anesthetic into his skin and muscles. Then I quickly scrubbed, put on sterile shoulder-length gloves and started to operate. It didn't take long to make the 10-inch incision, probe into his abdominal cavity and retract the diseased portion of gut. Sherman was snoring and lying quietly.

All we had to do now was to clamp off the intussusception with intestinal forceps, remove it, and then suture the healthy normal ends back together. Sounds simple. And it must be when the patient is completely out of it and is not liable to come up fighting at any moment.

However, just as I clamped, Sherman bellowed, strained and tried to raise his head. The result was a half bushel basket full of intestines delivered out of the incision into our hands.

"More Rompun!" I yelled as I stuffed intestines back into the abdominal cavity with panicky enthusiasm. There is a real art to replacing viscera back through an incision into its proper place. Often, you can be pushing and apparently making progress when you suddenly realize that, for each loop of gut that gets replaced, there are two loops that come back out. The novice simply cannot believe that a grown bull has only 150 feet of intestines. It seems like so much more.

Eventually, the viscera was replaced, the "bad" part removed and the two ends sutured back together. The muscles were sutured together with the heaviest catgut that I had available.

Raked tail through incision . . .

Just as I started to close the skin, his tail came loose from its tie and he raked the filthy thing through the incision. What else could possibly go wrong? Multiple flushings with sterile saline and penicillin helped restore the incision to at least visible cleanliness. The skin sutures were completed without great incident, although he was beginning to move his legs with greater enthusiasm.

We removed the restraining ropes, IV apparatus and, with the help of the few remaining hard-core helpers, set him up and removed all the head ropes. He just sat there half asleep, drooling profusely. He didn't look too badly at the moment, considering what he had been through. The next 12 to 24 hours would be critical, though, and perhaps by then we would know if he was going to survive or not.

As usual, the students had many questions to ask about the goings on of the last couple of hours.

"Sir," one began, "it seems to me that you weren't nearly sterile enough in technique; you should have scrubbed the incision three times instead of only two, and I noticed that you didn't change scalpels between skin and muscle. Why not?"

I tried not to bristle up as I quoted from some anonymous and brilliant sage.

"Son, when you are up to your gallowses in alligators, it's hard to remember that your initial objective was to drain the swamp!"

170

43

Sherman, Part IV

THE first 24 hours following surgery to correct a blocked intestine in an adult bovine seems to be the most critical period.

The suddenly-opened-up gut allows the backed-up and toxic material to flow freely past the newly sutured area and into the empty part below. This toxic material is absorbed by the cow and a toxic shock syndrome can be the result. The day or so following surgery usually finds the cow "painting the walls" with a black, smelly diarrhea.

Sherman was no exception. When I arrived at his stall the next day, I peered cautiously through a crack in the door. He was standing, which was a good sign, but he had his head pressed in the corner as if he had a terrific migraine headache. Sure enough, he had profuse diarrhea, as evidenced by the black, sticky straw on the floor and the streaky black walls.

"How's he doin', Keith?" I asked the student whom I had assigned as Sherman's personal aide.

"He's feeling right pert this morning," he replied, "pert enough that he won't let me get in there to clean up the stall."

"Well, if he's feeling that well, go ahead and put him in the chute and give him his treatments. Then you can clean up."

In the back of my mind, a little voice told me not to put him in the chute. As we coaxed Sherman out of the stall, the voice told me again, but I didn't listen as the big bull strode gingerly but briskly down the alleyway, around the corner and into the chute leading to the squeeze.

Since there was plenty of help, I decided to make a quick call to Mrs. Ramsey before getting into the activities of the day.

"He's doing as well as can be expected," I told her, as I heard the clanging of the chute. "It's just too early to tell which way he's going to go."

"Oh, I'm just so thankful," she said as she sniffed. I could almost hear the wringing of her hands. "Mr. Ramsey nor I either one slept a wink last night for worrying about Shermie."

"Well, don't worry . . ."

Just as I said "worry," Keith came running up, shouting and waving his arms.

"It's an emergency, Dr. John, it's a **big** emergency!"

"I'll call you back later, Mrs. Ramsey, it appears like we have some emergency that just drove up," I told her calmly as we said our goodbyes.

There's entrails everywhere . . .

"Naw, Doc, it's Sherman! He hit the side of the squeeze chute and ripped his incision wide open. There's entrails everywhere!"

"Oh, no! And with all this work to do!" I answered in dismay, as we raced to the scene of the ongoing chaos.

When we rounded the corner, we saw the big bull standing quietly with at least a number three washtub full of his abdominal contents hanging limply from a gaping hole in his side. The previous day's suture material, now broken and mangled, was sticking out of the jagged muscle fibers at crazy and useless angles. Few sights that I have ever seen, before or since, rivaled that one.

I knew that we had only two choices — immediate euthanasia or the immediate replacement of the digestive organs and resuturing the belly wall. I also knew that the former suggestion would not be acceptable to Mrs. Ramsey.

By now the students knew what to do, since it had been rehearsed. Suddenly, Rompun, a surgical pack, suture material of all types were thrust into the midst of the nightmarish scene. Rubber-gloved hands were carefully scrubbing skin, while others were gently washing fragile loops of intestines and keeping them moist. The suture line on the repaired gut looked great.

As the sedative took effect, we collapsed the side of the chute and gently rolled him out onto the floor, replaced the mass of bowels and started suturing from both ends of the incision. This time I was using a nonabsorbable material.

"Looks like well rope, it's so big," one good ol' boy drawled. "Bet that'll hold!"

After another hour of sewing, we had the job completed. So we propped the bull up on his sternum and discussed the situation.

"It'll be a wonder if that ol' rascal lives," uttered one student.

Too mean to die . . .

"Naw, he'll make it, 'cause he's just too mean to die," said another.

"If he does survive, I'm sure his incision line will get infected," I said carefully, "but we'll cross that creek when we get there."

With that pronouncement, we decided to have an early and quick lunch. Vienna sausages, moon pies and RC colas were devoured in short order. The cause of Sherman's problem, the survival rate and his future all were discussed. As we headed back, another student appeared.

"You know that ol' bull y'all been working on all morning?" he asked.

"What now?" we all asked in unison. We expected the worst.

"Well, he's standing up over there by the loading chute eatin' on a bale of wheat straw like he hasn't eaten in a week," he said.

Sherman survived. After that day he ate well, moved well and seemed fine, with one exception. His sutures became infected. On several occasions over the next several months, it was necessary for us to dig into the healed incision and remove sutures that acted as foreign bodies and caused the infection.

Veterinarians are called upon daily to perform difficult barnyard surgery on uncooperative and belligerent patients. I think most of us accept that challenge and do the best we can under the circumstances. It is often difficult for senior veterinary students to accept the fact that they may not be doing the ultra clean and aseptic surgery they read about in their textbooks and hear some of their white-smocked professors lecture about in the classroom.

173

Old Sherman did get infected, but he also survived, sired many calves after that, and gave Mr. and Mrs. Ramsey much pleasure as they watched him graze peacefully in his pasture.

Companion animals aren't always dogs, cats and horses, you know.

44

Vaccinating hogs in 10° weather

THE weather in the southern United States is tolerable — most of the time.

There are some people north of the Mason-Dixon line, though, who have the mistaken notion that it never gets cold in Alabama, Georgia or even Florida. The chamber of commerce of those sunbelt states might even perpetrate such erroneous thinking, but I can assure you that those same chamber folks never had vaccinated a drove of hogs around the middle of January when the weather is at its worst.

In fact, when I think about a classic example of misery and pain, I think of the time that Dr. Charles Otto of Langdale, Ala., and I were cordially invited to a hog cholera outbreak one January.

It was 10° above zero. The wind was slicing out of the northwest at 40 miles per hour and the humidity was 80 percent. Approximately 50 frozen swine carcasses that should have been sent to market the week before littered the lots. There were 50 more in the "thinking phase" of hog cholera and were at death's door, but just didn't know it yet.

Hogs don't think . . .

My professors and the veterinarians for whom I worked always told me that hogs were not supposed to think, so, when you saw one with his head down as if he were in deep meditative thought, then that hog had cholera for sure.

There were about 200 other swine of market size that were in apparent good health.

Our mission, if we decided to accept it, was to inject all swine that still were breathing with hog cholera antiserum. The dose of serum for a 150- to 200-pound hog was substantial, and more than one injection site would be required. We would be jabbing the shoats behind the ear, in the lower flank and/or in the loose skin of the armpit. Each beast would have to be captured and held, upside down, with his belly towards the vaccinator.

We had the services of four human hog catchers at our disposal. In addition to the two owners, there were two strapping boys, Ben and Wilbert, who were in their late teens and were cut from the "can snatcher" mold. Their biceps, although covered with a mass of flannel shirts, were approximately the size of M Farmall mufflers and were probably still thoroughly bronzed from last year's summer sun. Their forearms closely resembled sections of wagon tongues and could be seen quietly rippling in spite of their covering.

After a brief orientation as to how we were to proceed, Ben spoke up.

"Wilbert," he slowly drawled, "ye got 'ny chewin' terbackey?"

"I got muh britches on, ain't I?" retorted Wilbert, in the same identical drawl, as he tossed a pack towards his brother. He then loudly announced that he was ready to commence catching hogs.

Pants were hitched up, stocking caps reset, hands spit on, and the proceedings began.

In spite of the fact that many of the hogs were walking zombies, they still possessed the uncanny talent for evading the groping paws of the boys. When disturbed, some of the swine appeared to come alive and would avoid a would-be tackler by demonstrating a scatback type head fake which would leave Wilbert skidding to an icy stop in the opposite direction. As the hog would join a wad of his colleagues, he would look back over his shoulder at his human pursuers and appear to taunt them with a sneering grin.

Eventually, though, the porkers would meet their "Waterloo," as the boys did not give up easily. One would grab a flopping ear while the other would seize a rear leg in a vise grip type lock, and then they would easily turn the beast upside down for his turn with the serum needle.

Problems arose quickly however, because of the inclement weather. Hands, although covered with Jack 'n Jenny work gloves, soon became painfully frozen. Expressions of excruciating pain began to show on the ruddy faces of all participants.

"Hurry up, Doc!" Ben pleaded as he held a squirming Poland China, "My holt is slippin' on this here hog!"

I was trying to inject as fast as possible, but my hands were frozen, too. In addition, the old worn-out 40cc range type syringe that I was using leaked badly. When I withdrew serum from the 50cc bottle, some of the cold serum oozed down on my shaking hands and froze there. So my hands were in worse shape than theirs.

The low point of the day came when I vaccinated Wilbert by mistake. Somehow, the hog that he was holding wriggled as I jabbed, and the half-inch, 15-gauge needle sunk softly into a meaty human thigh, up to the hub.

"OW, OW, OW!" Wilbert screamed, "You've shot me in the laig, Doc!"

He was hopping around on one leg, like a jumping jack, holding his vaccinated leg up in the air.

"I'm ruint!" he squalled, as he hopped into a group of scattering porcines, "My laig's gonna fall off from this here cholery!"

In light of the events, we all decided that a brief intermission was called for. The owners quickly built a roaring old tire fire outside the barn, and we tried our best to warm our stiff and numb hands and toes.

Wilbert was giving me a wide berth by now, and was constantly mumbling and massaging the site of the vaccination accident on his massive leg. If I walked around behind him, he turned all the way around, too, just so he could keep an eye on me and that needle.

"Do ye feel like you're turnin' into a hog yet, Wilbert!" Ben said, among thigh-slapping laughter.

"Reckon Doc'll charge you for that shot?" needled Ben.

"You shut up, Ben!" Wilbert whined, "or I'll bus' you open!"

This brotherly exchange was greeted by more laughter from all the other participants, except me. I had never vaccinated a human being against cholera before, and I didn't know what would happen to that human leg. I could envision all sorts of bad things happening. First, the leg would swell badly, then gangrene would set in, then a long hospital stay would culminate in loss of the leg.

I quickly shook my head to clear it of those ridiculous thoughts. Surely to goodness, nothing would happen to old Wilbert's leg!

The rest of the vaccinations eventually were completed in icy misery. When we finally trudged out of the manure-and-frozen-corn-cob-covered lot, Wilbert and Ben were complaining about the difficulty of the just-completed task.

"That work's so hard, I wouldn't do it for $60 a week!" declared Ben.

"Me neither!" I said to myself, "me neither!"

I met Wilbert on the street about a month later. He was going at a canter and showed no signs of lameness. When he spied me, he stopped in his tracks, then quickly crossed the street, all the time looking warily backwards in my direction. I sure was relieved to see that cholera had not taken him away!

45

"Nice cow you got there"

My DAD had called and asked me to be on the lookout for a new bull for his small herd of Angus cows. His present herd consists of descendants of the Jersey cows we used to milk by hand during "the war."

About the time I had left home for ag school, Mr. Liggett, our A.I. man, had bred the Jerseys to good black bulls, and thus a good milking herd of black beef cows was established. Today, as a "real" cattleman, Dad can feel justified in driving around in a muddy red pickup truck with a gun rack over the rear window, a shepherd dog riding in the back and baler twine hanging out the tailgate — that is, if he wants to.

"You see a lot of cattle in your rounds," he had said over the phone. "See if you can locate me a nice, young, high-powered, forage-tested, gentle, black bull that will sire small calves that grow fast and won't have pink eye."

"You don't want much, do you?" I had kidded him.

"Oh yeah, I almost forgot," he added, "I don't want to pay much for him either."

Now where was I going to find the perfect bull that also was inexpensive? I commenced my search in midsummer by reading all the cattlemen's journals, talking to all my cowboy buddies and scanning all the pastures as I made my rounds in the northern part of the state.

Named him Herschel . . .

Finally, about the first of November, I found him at a certified performance test sale and bought him at a reasonable price. A friend trailered him to another friend's house for boarding until I could pick him up. I named him Herschel. I borrowed my friend Claude's four-wheel drive Ford and stock trailer one Saturday in early December, loaded Herschel up and pointed the truck in a northwest direction.

When I reached Atlanta, the fun began. Have you ever driven through the big city and all its impatient traffic, pulling livestock behind you? The dumb, open-mouthed stares from passers-by, the little kids in back seats pointing fingers at the "odd" animal creature and pedestrians holding their noses are just some of the interesting sights that you may see.

When I stopped for gas, the attendant saw Herschel and started an interesting conversation.

"Nice cow you got there," he allowed.

"Well it's actually a bull, not a cow," I corrected.

"What's the difference?" he queried.

"Cows are females and bulls are males," I explained.

"Oh," he said, somewhat perplexed. "Are you gonna eat him?"

"No, I'll put him with some cows, he'll breed them and then they'll have little calves next year."

"Yeah, yeah, I got it now," he said happily. "Then they'll make milk, and you'll take it to the dairy store and sell it!"

"Well, no, that's dairy cows. We're talking about beef cows." I knew that it was a lost cause, so I eased into the store for a cold carton. How can you explain beef cattle production to someone who is a livestock production illiterate?

The next pause was at a rest stop at the state line. I was back at the trailer checking on Herschel and chatting with him about the weather when a new Mercedes diesel chattered up and parked beside us. Out climbed a middle-aged person resembling a male, dressed in the latest and most expensive casual wear. He wore several neck chains, had multiple rings on his fingers and had large Polaroid sunglasses perched on his nose.

"Hey, man, nice cow you got there," he pronounced, as he placed both hands on the trailer and peeked in between the slats. At the same instant, Herschel stuck his large, messy nose in the same spot and snorted viciously.

The neck-chain-clad stranger reeled backwards and ricocheted off the right rear fender of his peach-colored luxury car.

"Hey, man," he whined as he looked down at the expensive shirt Herschel had used as a handkerchief, "you didn't tell me he was so rude and uncouth!"

"He's not," I giggled. "He just needed to blow his nose right then. Here, I've got a rag under the front seat that we can use to wipe your shirt off."

"No, not with that filthy thing," he screamed. "Do you know what this shirt cost me?" He was flicking at the spots on it now with his pinkie. About every third flick he would reach down and rub the peachy Mercedes, looking for an obscure scratch. When he jogged toward the washroom, Herschel and I vamoosed.

An hour or two later, we pulled up to McDonald's for lunch. The mechanical device where you order for take-out service was out of order, so we drove right up to the window.

Ordered alfalfa . . .

"Let me have a Big Mac, a large thing of fries and two milks, please," I ordered. "And let me have some alfalfa for my partner in the back."

I could see the young lady's puzzled facial expression as she covered up the microphone and mumbled something to the chunky-looking manager.

"Sir, I'm sorry," she apologized, "we don't have any alfalfa sprouts, but we do have some fresh cole slaw."

"No, I think he wants hay," I said as I pointed to the rear.

"Oh, it's a horsey," she squealed. "You were just kidding me!"

"Well, he's actually a mean Mexican fightin' bull, but I guess he does look a little like a chubby horsey," I allowed with eyes closed.

Two or three minutes later, I had my burger in hand and was driving off.

"Bye, horsey," cooed the girl.

"Moo," said Herschel.

When I got back on the road, I tried to analyze the three situations that Herschel and I had just experienced.

Why is it that some people don't know the difference between bulls and cows, beef and dairy animals, bulls and horses, or what all these animals do for them? In addition, those same people have no earthly idea about the habits, husbandry and dining requirements of those animals or why farm animals are so important to the health and well-being of all people. Does the young lady who served up my burger, fries and milk ever stop and wonder where all that good food comes from, how accessible it is and how inexpensive it all is?

I finally came up with the answer. Food producers actually are being penalized for their own efficiency and their ability to produce large amounts of high-quality food. The man at the service station and the freaky guy in the peach Mercedes probably never have milked a cow, wrung a chicken's neck, rendered out lard or dug potatoes. They and millions of other nonfarm dwellers definitely would have a better appreciation for the food supply chain if they were required to spend an active, working year on a real farm.

Finally, I arrived at Dad's farm, backed up to the pasture gate and turned Herschel out with the cows. They stopped grazing fescue in midchew and raised their heads in wonder as he galloped out to introduce himself.

"Did you have a good trip up?" Dad asked.

"Yes, sir, it was a most educational trip," I answered. "Old Herschel is 'cityfied' now, as well as certified!"

Do you suppose it will take a famine in the land before people will understand and appreciate their quality food, how little it costs and the few who toil so hard to produce it?

46

"You gon' play tennis or dehorn cows?"

IT WAS a nice October day in my first year of veterinary practice when I had my first bird patient crisis.

"What a pretty little parakeet!" I allowed, as the elderly lady placed the cage upon the exam table.

The little fellow was kind of an iridescent mixed green color even though his feathers were ruffled and askew. He was sitting quietly in the bottom of the cage with his head hanging low. It appeared that he was staring at the cage floor contemplating a terrific headache.

"Yes sir, Doctor, Buster's been doing poorly for the last couple of days," she said. "He's not his usual chirping and vibrant self. He just sits there acting like he's cold all the time."

"Well, let's see what we can do about that," I suggested, as I opened the cage door and reached inside.

I quickly captured the feathery creature in my meaty right fist and was extracting him from his home when my attention was temporarily drawn to a loud noise in the opposite direction. It was only two dogs involved in a fracas in the kennel area.

"Heah, you dogs!" I yelled, "Quieten down in there! Sit!"

Immediate silence prevailed. It's amazing sometimes how intimidating a loud voice can be.

I had almost forgotten about the little bird in my right hand until I felt his beak flop weakly onto my forefinger. At first I thought that maybe he was experiencing a "falling out" spell. Remembering back to the avian medicine courses that I had taken recently in veterinary school, nothing computed regarding fainting poultry, however. At that moment, I was pretty sure that I had just bought into the bird business.

"What's wrong with Buster, Doctor?" the poor lady asked. I noticed that her eyes had widened and her mouth was gaped open in apparent shock. I realized that my face was frozen with the same look of restrained panic.

"Uh, why I believe he's passed out" I stammered. "Let me see if I can give him CPR!"

I quickly laid Buster out on the cold exam table and made heroic efforts to revive him. Although CPR in a wee bird is quite difficult, I made a valiant attempt. I tried mouth-to-beak resuscitation, chest massage and loud talk. None of that worked. I tossed him into the deep freeze for three seconds in hopes that the brief severe cold would initiate respiratory action. That didn't work either. He was dead.

Buster was dead . . .

"I'm afraid Buster had a massive heart attack, Ma'am." I said slowly. "Unfortunately, it was fatal."

"Oh, no!" cried the lady, "poor little Buster! He never hurt anybody. Oooh, oooh!"

The poor lady was sobbing now as she cradled the little bird in her hands. Her heart was breaking.

I was looking around for some strong rope and a chair since I was considering hanging myself from the rafters. My gaze fell upon the scalpels on the counter, and I wondered if it would be more expedient to just slash my wrists. I really felt rotten.

"I am truly sorry about Buster," I apologized, "but sometimes these little birds just go into shock and die when they are stressed. Perhaps we can find another one somewhere."

"No, I just wish you had been a little more gentle with him. You deal with big animals most of the time, and you are just too rough on little birds," she lectured, between sobs and tears.

"And another thing," she continued. "If you are going to work with people's beloved pets, you should wear some nice slacks, a tie and a white jacket. You must look like a doctor!"

What more could I say? I really had not been that rough with him, other than yelling at the dogs. That loud racket probably had done him in. And, my appearance *could* have been improved.

I looked down at my big, rough hands. They were calloused and stained with black tattoo ink, were cracked, cut and chapped from rough farm work. No wonder the poor lady was disturbed. They surely didn't look like "bird-healing" hands.

Within an hour, I had changed my appearance and was on my way to dehorn some rough-looking, line-backed, piney-woods cows. I still was shaken from the bird incident but was vowing that, from that time on, I would be more gentle with my patients *and* do something about my hands and wearing apparel.

The cowboy crowd at the corral looked like escapees from the mean farm. None of them had shaved in days, and they all wore scowls that would have stopped Superman in his tracks. They looked at me in disgust as they jawed their chews of tobacco.

"Another green vetnerry!" one mumbled between spits. "Got on pretty white coveralls and little white tennis shoes! And look at the lily white hands!"

"Doc, you gon' play tennis or dehorn cows?" another toothless wonder questioned amid laughter, snickering and spitting.

"Look," I said, "one of y'all just come up here and catch heads for me, and I'll get these horns removed. Don't worry about my appearance."

Within minutes we had a head caught, the nose tonged and pulled around to the side. The cow was one of about 30 or so aged cows whose horns were long, with numerous concentric rings, and were the consistency of antique granite. I gently lifted the heavy Keystone dehorners and placed them meticulously over the horn, making sure the cut would include a ring of hair all the way around the base of the horn. Then I slowly tried to pull the handles together. The cow bellowed, stomped in the chute and slung her head as I strained, squenched my eyes closed and gritted my teeth. But the horn remained intact.

Too gentle . . .

"Looka here, Doc!" the head cowboy yelled, "you're just too easy and gentle! You act like this is one of your lit-tle lap dogs or a sick canary. You got to go at this hard and kind of vicious-like! Here, lemme show you how we do this back home in Texas!"

With that, he elbowed me aside, grabbed the two han-dles, and with a karate-type yell, snatched the two handles together. The immediate result was a loud lightning-like crack, followed quickly by a deafening cow bellow and geysering of blood which covered the front of my attire.

"That's how it's done, young feller!" the pleased cowboy uttered, as he rendered the air greenish-brown with a sudden irrigation of well-used tobacco juice.

There certainly was nothing gentle about the way he removed the horn from that cow! As I gently tried to pull the bleeding artery, the cowboy continued his critique of my technique and appearance.

"Doc, you don't do much cow work do you? Yo' hands are too pretty and clean! If you're gonna go out onto the farm and git amongst 'em, you oughta wear some work clothes and boots. Them whites just won't do!"

"Yeah, that's right," echoed another member of the crew. "We had one vet come out here with a tie on! A tie!! I can't believe it!"

Veterinarians engaged in mixed practices often have a tough time making all their clients happy with their appearance, wardrobe selection and the condition of their hands. Also, it's kind of hard to work all day with a wild, unruly herd of Brahman cattle, then come back to the clinic and adjust to fragile birds and kittens.

With this in mind, I have four pieces of advice for young, inexperienced veterinarians who have entered mixed practices.

First, do not examine and treat sick and fragile parakeets immediately after vaccinating and/or dehorning a herd of cows.

Second, owners presenting sick parakeets for treatment should be requested to remove the bird from the cage themselves and to restrain it while you make the examination. It will save you considerable embarrassment, and it will save those owners a lot of birds!

Third, wear whatever you want to; just try to be clean! Dress for the occasion!

Fourth, use plenty of Bag Balm, or Cornhusker's Lotion on your rough hands. It is okay to use ladies sweet-smelling hand lotion in a pinch; just don't let the cowboys find out about it!

47

A strange Christmas day call

Doc, I hate to bother you, it bein' Christmas and all," the early morning caller said, "but one of my neighbors has this here cow and everything's come out of 'er!"

It was Carney Sam Jenkins, the local self-made cow doctor. I could always recognize his telephone voice with ease, since he always talked real loud and used his best English.

I also knew that Carney Sam didn't mind calling me at any time of the day or night, Christmas, birthday or even at little league ball game time. The reason he usually called was that he had gotten himself in over his head and needed help, some equipment or an instrument that I had. At least he knew what his limitations were and asked for help before he got beyond the point of no return on the cow or mule or whatever. Lots of my clients didn't know when to stop and get assistance, so they just went blindly on until they killed their patient.

"Is she prolapsed, Carney Sam?" I asked. "Did she calve during the night?"

"Yeah, yeah, Doc, it's her womb awright," he excitedly related. "Looks like at least a shuck basket full of stuff hangin' out. It jus' don't look like it's gonna go back in. You just got to come and hope us out!"

"Well, whose cow is it?"

"Junior Mears, Doc. You know him, he's back there in the woods on the left side of the road just before you git to Miss Ruby's store. By the way, Doc, that thing's tore up pretty bad."

When he said "Junior Mears," I knew that it was going to be bad. Most people in the community called him by his nickname, "Brimmer" Mears, since he owned a herd of wild Brahman cattle. He had a general idea of how many cows he owned, but they were so wild it was practically

187

impossible to get them out of the woods, corraled and counted.

When we had tested for brucellosis, it had taken several horses and riders, four of the meanest "catch" dogs ever bred and a brand new 8-foot-tall catch pen made of creosoted 2 by 10 lumber. Even then it had taken several days of work to get the 200 or so head penned and tested. Most of the cows could leap like gazelles, yet they were mean as riled rattlesnakes.

Brimmer Mears made whiskey back in the woods where his cows roamed. It was said by tasting experts that his product was superb, and it was also said that he had customers who drove many miles to gladly trade a $20 bill for a gallon of the crystal clear liquid.

He was also an accomplished whittler. He was always carving on pieces of wood while sitting at Miss Ruby's store, and those plain, ordinary blocks of wood were magically transformed by his pocket knife into elegant carvings of little horses, or cows or deer. Our three children often rode with me on calls, and they had admired his creations at Miss Ruby's store. He was a rough individual who had much artistic talent, but he didn't even know it.

She's a mite fractious . . .

"Well, have you tried to get the thing back in?" I asked.

"Actually Doc, we ain't been able to get our hands on 'er yet. She's just a mite fractious. But we're gonna try real hard to git her in the catch pen fo' you git here!"

I peeked through the curtains to see a cold, overcast and gloomy Christmas day being tormented by a piercing and persistent drizzle. Few things are much worse on man or beast than 35° southern rain. Just thinking about stripping to the waist in an icy pasture and struggling with a reluctant prolapse and a protesting patient was enough to send shivers through my bones.

"I'll swear, Carney Sam," I exclaimed, "you're gonna get me out there in all this misery and mud, and we'll spend all Christmas day runnin' after a fool cow that's wilder'n a March hare . . ."

"Naw, naw, we'll git 'er in the pen lack I said, and you can tho' yo' rope on her neck when she runs by. I seen you use zat lariat over to the sale barn the other day. You're really good with that thing!" he bragged. I knew that I was being had.

"Tell you what, Carney," I negotiated, "my in-laws are here for Christmas. Let us open up our few presents and let the young 'uns see what old Santy brought 'em, and then I'll come on out about 10. How's that?"

I could hear him conversing with Brimmer, with his hand over the phone's mouthpiece.

"Brimmer said that'd be awright, Doc. He said to not forget to bring yo' rope."

As I sat and watched the kids playing with their new toys and plunging their little hands down into goodie-stuffed stockings, I heard Jan and her mother conversing.

"Does he get paid time and a half or double time for working on holidays?" her mother asked.

"No, Mother," Jan replied. "We're real lucky if he just gets time!"

At 9:30 I sprinted through the punishing rain to my truck parked under the tall pine trees, cranked up the sluggish engine and splashed out the driveway. The rain hinted of freezing on the windshield as I aimed the Chevy in the general direction of Carney Sam, Brimmer and the ill-mannered cow.

Going through the small town, I saw the homes dressed out in their seasonal finery. Colored lights around front doors, windows and draped over and through cedar trees in living room picture windows blinked out their happy greetings. Strange cars with out-of-state license tags signaled that Junior or Sis had come home from the big city for the holiday and had parked their crammed-full autos in their old parking spots. I wondered how many of the people in those warm homes had ever heard of a prolapse.

A few minutes later I was turning into Brimmer Mears' narrow driveway. Actually, it wasn't a driveway at all, it was an old dry creek bed. Rocks of all sizes were imbedded in the concrete-like slippery clay, and this required slow going for the half mile to the dilapidated shack that Brimmer called home.

The shack was nothing more than an old, one-room structure where cotton was once stored until it was taken to the gin. You could see underneath the shack, all the way through, since it had no underpinning. Six or eight frazzled and wet dogs tore out from under the house as my truck shook and rattled up. As they barked and bit at the tires, a fight broke out between two blue tick hounds, since there weren't enough tires to go around.

Suddenly the door flew open and a rough-looking, un-shaven Brimmer yelled loudly at the dogs. It was obvious-ly a much practiced ritual.

"Heah! You dogs git away from that feller's truck," he screamed. With that pronouncement, he reached down, grabbed a rock the size of a prune and expertly hurled it, catching one of the curs right between the eyes. The dog blinked, slinked and staggered back underneath the house, while the remainder of the pack tucked their heads and tails sheepishly and hid behind bushes, trees, the woodpile and the junk cars that were up on blocks in the front yard. Carney Sam's old doorless Dodge truck was there, too, backed up on a bank, ready for a quick getaway. Actually, his battery was perpetually weak, so he always had to park the thing on a hill in order to "roll start" it.

Presently, Carney Sam joined Brimmer at the shack's door. They were pulling on more shirts, pants, vests and denim jumpers over their long-handled clad carcasses. All these extra clothes were indicated, since the weather seemed to be taking a turn for the worse. Sleet was be-ginning to mix with the rain now, and a glaze was forming on the pine and cedar trees.

"Where's the cow, Carney?" I asked.

"Rat down yonder amongst them woods," he an-nounced. "We can drive rat up to 'er Doc, and you can jus' drop that rope on 'er."

If I had a dollar for every time I've heard that phrase, I'd be financially secure for life.

"Doc, since I got this four-wheel-drive jeep le's jes' all ride in it," said Brimmer.

As I got in beside them, I caught the strong odor of moon-shine whiskey. Obviously the two men had been charging themselves with some of Brimmer's homemade antifreeze before they ventured back out with the patient. I was glad that we hadn't taken my truck, since the odor of that whis-key penetrated truck interiors and stayed there for months.

We made small talk about the bad weather and cow

prices as we nervously hung onto our seats. Brimmer was hitting stumps and running over small saplings as he made a straight line toward the cow. As we came closer, I could see that she was a spotted first-calf Brahman heifer with horns sufficiently long for professional goring.

She went into a canter when she saw us, and about every four step she would kick viciously at the large, shredded gelatin-like mass hanging from her rear parts when it slapped and tickled her hocks. The prolapse was unrecognizable as a body organ, since it had been kicked, dragged through thickets and now almost frozen. It was beyond saving. If we could catch the beast, it looked like our only alternative would be to amputate.

"Get as close to her as you can, Brimmer," I shouted, "and I'll try to rope her."

After several passes with the jeep, the heifer stopped and challenged the vehicle's right front fender. I luckily dropped the rope over her horns, jumped out of the vehicle, streaked for the nearest tree and quickly took two loops around it with the long end just as she streaked past me, heading for the safety of the freezing creek.

When she reached the end of the nylon rope, she was suddenly snatched backwards like a rodeo calf. But while the cow stopped dead still, the mangled organ quickly became dislodged from its bodily attachments and continued on its way to the creek, soaring through the trees in arc-like aerial flight until it fell into the creek with a splash.

Meanwhile, the potent alcoholic potions that my two colleagues had consumed earlier had taken effect, and they were having trouble exiting the vehicle and walking upright. Finally, they arrived on the scene just as I was examining the south end of the cow.

"Carney Sam, looka here! This man's done put a healin' on this cow!" slurred Brimmer as he smiled and pointed at the patient.

"Doc, how'd you git t'at thang back in'are so fast?" asked Carney Sam, as he tried to focus his eyes.

"Just a trick I learned in school," I retorted. "Don't take long if you know what you're doin'."

I quickly injected her with some "wonderful drug," as Carney called it, got the two men back to the jeep and then released the heifer. I reckon that she had fought enough, so she just trotted back out into the rocky pasture, turned and looked at me, then disappeared over the hill.

Carney Sam and Brimmer were in the jeep arguing over who was going to drive. Both were on the verge of moderate intoxication.

"Move over, both of you. I'm driving this machine!" I ordered. They quickly obeyed and inched over in the seat.

The return trip back to the shack took longer with me driving, even though I was freezing to death. The brutal wind was whistling through cracks, holes and rips in the roof, and the freezing rain was dripping down on my ears and neck.

"Brimmer, you better sell that cow before long, 'cause I doubt if she'll ever have another calf," I said, with tongue in cheek and with fingers crossed. I didn't think that either man could understand what had really happened to the cow in the past 30 minutes. At least not at present. Perhaps later, after their overworked livers had cleared the toxic alcohol from their systems.

When we finally arrived at the shack, Brimmer was sober enough to ask me into the house to wash up. As I poured hot water from the kettle into a wash pan and then scrubbed with Lava soap, Brimmer disappeared outside for a few minutes. Carney Sam and I conversed about how doctors never get off for Christmas or other holidays and how little they got paid for their services.

While I was drying on an old feed sack towel, Brimmer walked unsteadily in the house.

"What I owe ye, Doc?" he slurred as he pulled a huge wad of greenbacks out of a crinkled paper sack. I knew it was moonshine money, but I also knew that the grocery store guy and the bank accepted it just like it was church offering.

"Aw, just peel me off $20 worth and we'll be square," I said.

"Doc, I put a box in the back of yo' truck," Brimmer said. "You might check on it when you git to the house. I hope yo' young 'uns enjoy their Santy Claus!"

On the way home my curiosity got the best of me, so I stopped on the roadside, got out in the slush and opened up the back of the truck. There beside the gallons of worm medicine and the calf jack sat a big box. Looking inside, I

192

saw two half gallons of Brimmer's homemade whiskey. It was so clear and shiny, and it beaded up when shook. Also in the box were two gallons of sorghum syrup and three little wooden, hand-carved Brahman cows. They were beautiful. It must have taken days to produce them.

Driving home, I thought about the strange man, Brimmer Mears, and his inconsistencies. He was rough as a cob, and he made, sold and drank illegal whiskey. He lived in a one-room shack at the end of a nearly impossible "road" and owned an unknown number of unbelievably wild cows. Yet he possessed considerable talent for producing wood carvings and often gave them away to children.

They kids loved their little wooden cows, Jan and I sopped the syrup with her good homemade biscuits, but I did not consume the alcohol. I gave one jug away to a desperate friend and used the other to start charcoal fires.

There are all sorts of interesting people in a veterinarians' life.